THE VEGAN COOKBOOK FOR ATHLETES

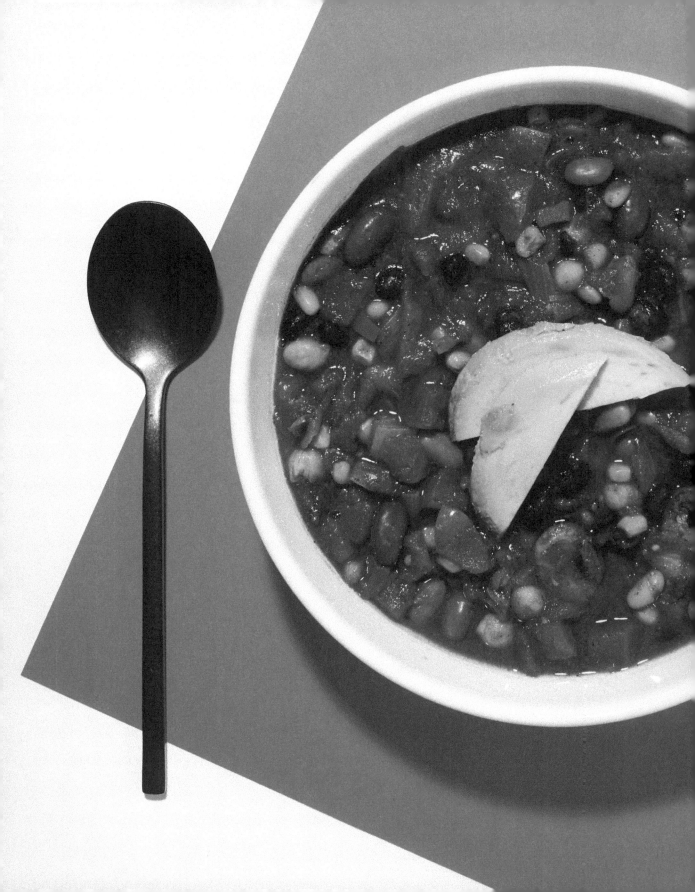

THE VEGAN COOKBOOK FOR ATHLETES

101 Recipes and 3 Meal Plans to Build Endurance and Strength

ANNE-MARIE CAMPBELL

ROCKRIDGE
PRESS

For general information on our other products and services or to obtain technical support, please contact our Customer Care Department within the United States at (866) 744-2665, or outside the United States at (510) 253-0500.

Rockridge Press publishes its books in a variety of electronic and print formats. Some content that appears in print may not be available in electronic books, and vice versa.

TRADEMARKS: Rockridge Press and the Rockridge Press logo are trademarks or registered trademarks of Callisto Media Inc. and/or its affiliates, in the United States and other countries, and may not be used without written permission. All other trademarks are the property of their respective owners. Rockridge Press is not associated with any product or vendor mentioned in this book.

Interior and Cover Designer: Carlos Esparza
Art Producer: Megan Baggott
Editor: Jed Bickman
Production Editor: Ruth Sakata Corley

Cover and pp. 56, 74, 102, 124, 160, 172: Photography © 2020 Paul Sirisalee. Food styling by Kimberley Sirisalee.

pp. vi, 20, 54: Photography © Johnny Autry/Emulsion Studio, p. viii: Marija Vidal, p. xii: Amy Johnson, p. 2: Thomas J. Story, p. 30: Darren Muir, p. 186: Biz Jones.

Author photo courtesy of: Linda Estep

ISBN: Print 978-1-64739-018-1 | eBook 978-1-64739-019-8

R0

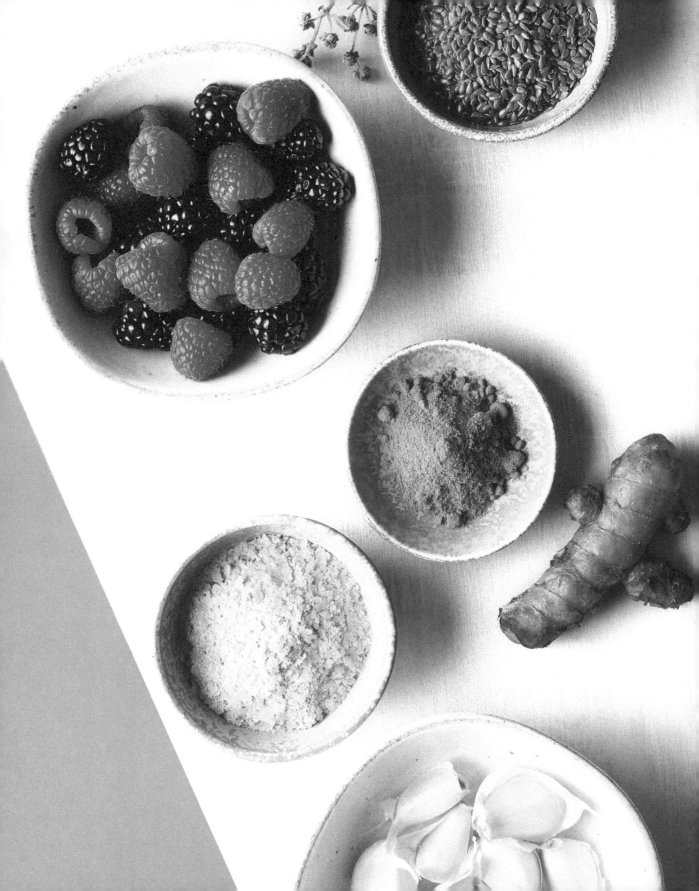

Contents

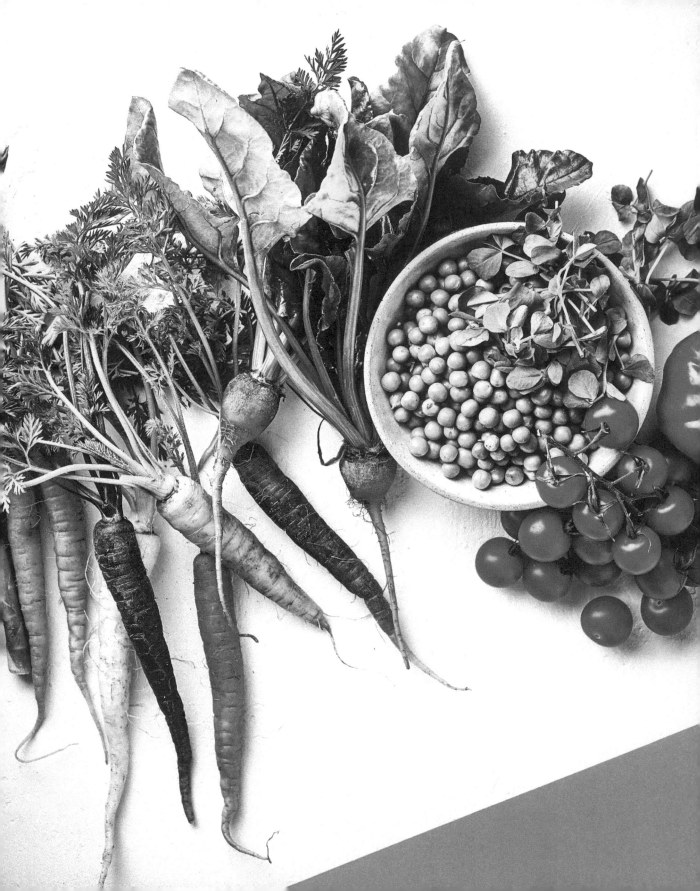

Introduction

As athletes, we're always looking for new ways to elevate our performance. More energy, quicker recovery, better sleep, and sharper mental focus are all critical for athletes. Whether you're vegan or veg-curious, this book will tell you how and why the vegan lifestyle is beneficial for athletes of all levels, ages, genders, and sports. Plant-based foods offer an abundance of nutrients and provide our bodies with all our essential needs, without the need for meat, dairy, or eggs.

Knowing what an athlete should eat can be confusing. There is a lot of conflicting information out there, and it can be hard to make sense of it all, especially when misinformation about protein, carbs, and athletic performance is widespread.

My journey as a competitive athlete started almost three decades ago, beginning with gymnastics, then ice hockey, and over the past 10 years, martial arts. I have trained in several martial arts, including Tae Kwon Do, Brazilian Jiu Jitsu, Muay Thai, and MMA. I am currently a black belt in Tae Kwon Do, with a record of 8–0 in competition.

I wasn't raised in a vegan household. I grew up with meals that mostly centered around meat and other animal-based products. When I was young and competing in gymnastics, I never really thought about nutrition or about how the foods I ate affected my performance. When I turned 16, I traded my spandex for skates and started playing ice hockey. During this time I started to become more aware of how different foods affected my energy levels, recovery, and asthma. I started to become an intuitive eater, meaning that I started to become highly attuned to how different foods affected how I felt, how much energy I had before hitting the wall, the speed of my recovery, the efficiency of my digestion, and the clarity of my mental focus. This was the key period in my life that sparked my passion for nutrition and holistic health.

During this time, I stopped eating beef, lamb, and pork. I had noticed that I did not digest those foods well, and they did nothing to increase my energy, endurance, or recovery. This was before we had endless amounts of information at our fingertips on the internet, so I spent a lot of time at the library researching and gaining a better understanding of the human body and its nutritional needs.

As I progressed into playing hockey at a competitive level, my performance was critical. I wanted to be a strong contributor on the team, and I felt an added pressure to perform, more so than during my years competing in the solo sport of gymnastics, in which I was the only one responsible for my place on the podium. Hockey players were getting faster, stronger, and more skilled. I had the ability to score as a forward, but I always struggled to find the right meals to give me the energy I needed to sustain me until the end of the game.

Jump ahead several years. I was looking for a sport to keep me active in the hockey off-season, and I found Tae Kwon Do. Shortly after starting to practice martial arts, I saw a post on social media about an undercover investigation into the treatment of animals on a farm. I clicked on the article and was horrified by what I saw. Until that moment, I had never thought about where my food came from. I always considered myself an animal lover, but I was disconnected from the reality of how the food I was eating got to my plate and what those animals had to endure. That was the start of my journey to the vegan lifestyle. I started by going vegetarian for 30 days. Within a few months, I made the full transition to vegan, veganizing my favorite meals and swapping out animal products for plant-based versions. The transition was easier than I expected, and it felt good to know my actions were now more ethically aligned with my beliefs.

While in the process of going vegan, I was training for my Tae Kwon Do black belt testing. Even though I made the switch to veganism for the animals, I was excited to see that I was experiencing health and performance benefits.

I had no problem passing my black belt test as a meat-free athlete, and I've never looked back!

At the dojo and at the hockey rink, people began to ask me what I was eating. They saw me full of energy and thriving as a vegan athlete and they were genuinely curious. That inspired me to start my website, MeatFreeAthlete.com, with the goal of documenting my journey, sharing recipes, giving lifestyle tips, spotlighting vegan athletes around the world, building community, and helping people go (or stay) vegan.

Continually expanding my knowledge is always a priority for me. Being a longtime holistic health advocate, I earned my Plant-Based Nutrition Certificate at the T. Colin Campbell Center for Nutrition Studies in partnership with eCornell University, which provides science-based education and truly empowers people to elevate their understanding of health and nutrition.

I've been vegan since 2011, and I continue to experience the benefits of having more energy than I had before. I train longer, feel stronger, maintain muscle more easily, and recover faster. My asthma has also improved significantly; I haven't used my inhaler in years. Most people just don't realize how good our bodies are meant to feel!

Sharing what I have learned over the past three decades is part of my mission to help people successfully transition to the vegan lifestyle. I am passionate about living a compassionate lifestyle and showing you the power of plant-based nutrition.

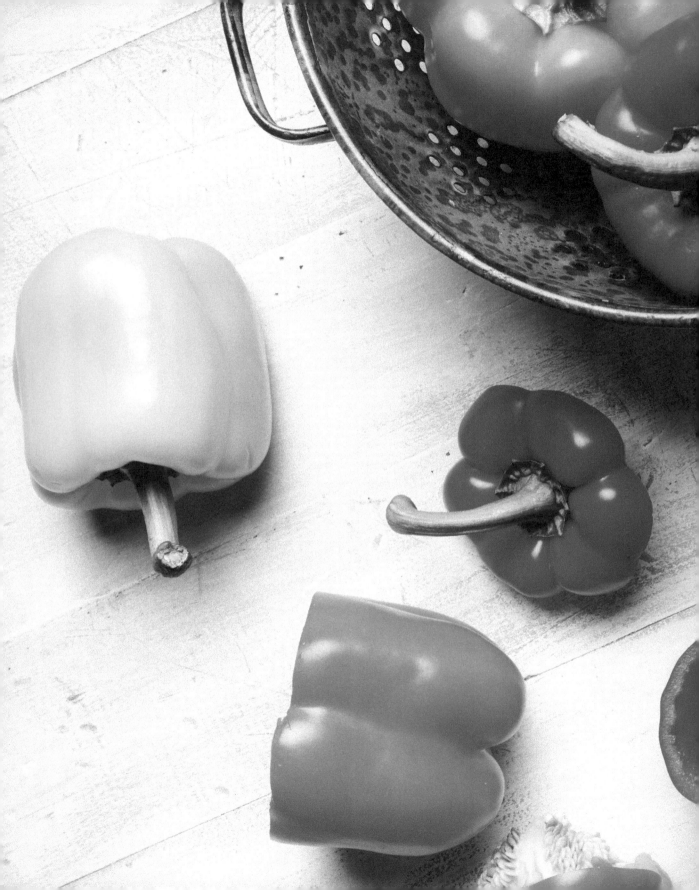

PART 1

Plant-Powered Performance

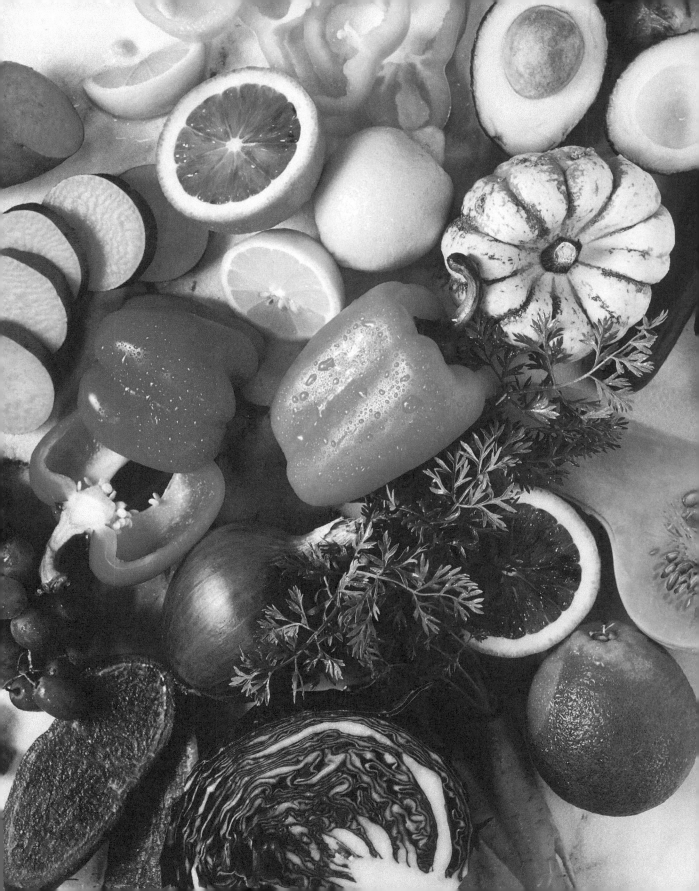

CHAPTER 1

Plant-Based Support for Your Specific Athletic Needs

A growing number of professional and Olympic athletes in various sports are thriving as vegans and competing at the highest levels. No matter what your level, you can ditch animal products and reach your potential. This chapter dives into the benefits athletes can gain from going vegan, and will help you understand your body's nutritional requirements, which foods to eat, and how to calculate your individual needs.

Being a great athlete isn't just about the workout, the training, or the game. How we fuel ourselves is a huge factor in success and longevity in our sport. Physical and mental health cannot be fully achieved without proper nutrition. Consistent training and eating the right foods must work together, with a focus on your personal goals and needs always at the forefront.

Flip the Script

It seems that despite the long and rapidly expanding list of professional vegan athletes, some people still fall back on the old stereotype that great athletic performance requires you to eat meat. Old beliefs often die hard. We all grew up hearing the same things about meat and dairy at school, on TV, and online, so it takes a conscious effort, as well as an open mind, to unlearn old ideas and learn new truths.

If you've started your vegan journey, have you been looking to find good sources of protein? Are you confused about how to balance your macronutrients to meet your athletic needs? Do you find yourself the target of teasing from people at your gym or on your team for trying the plant-based lifestyle? If you answered yes to any of the above, you are not alone. Rest assured, it is common for people to feel unsure at first, because there is a learning curve involved in going vegan and remaining athletically competitive.

The good news is that it is absolutely possible to make the transition to a vegan diet when you're an athlete, and you can get all the nutrition your body needs without sacrificing your performance. Countless vegan athletes all around the world are helping bust stereotypes daily within their own communities. No matter what your sport of choice, you can crush your goals as a vegan if you put in the work and persist.

No, You Don't Need Meat

The belief that meat is necessary for gaining muscle, staying lean, and being a great athlete is quickly becoming a thing of the past. The general public is starting to embrace the nutritional benefits of a balanced plant-based lifestyle, and it's not hard to find science to back up the advantages. Athletes of all levels are proving they can not only make the switch successfully but also thrive while doing so.

Nutrient density of a food is a key factor when looking at overall nutrition and protein quality. For example, meat can generally be a high-protein option, but it contains fewer of the other nutrients, which often makes it the weaker option compared with its plant-based protein counterpart.

Tofu, for example, has significantly higher amounts of essential nutrients such as calcium, iron, zinc, magnesium, and folate than chicken, according to the USDA FoodData Central. These essential nutrients are necessary for maintaining good health and are especially important for athletes because they help increase performance output because of the vital role they play in the optimal functioning and recovery of an active body.

Protein is not just one type of food; it is a nutrient made up of a combination of 20 amino acids. We can naturally produce 11 amino acids from chemicals already in our body; these are called nonessential amino acids. The remaining nine amino acids must be obtained from the foods we eat; these are called essential amino acids.

There is a misconception that plant-based protein sources are incomplete, meaning that they lack some essential amino acids. The truth is, all plants contain all essential amino acids, in varying amounts, as confirmed by Dr. John A. McDougall, a nutrition expert and the founder of the McDougall Foundation. So, the question then becomes, where do you get your amino acids? Because plant-based foods vary in their amino acid profiles, it is always best to eat a wide variety of foods. Not only is this a surefire way to get your essential aminos, but it is also a good way to reap the benefits of eating a variety of the nutrients that are plentiful in plants. We will continue our discussion of amino acids on page 13.

The Good, the Bad, the Science

Going vegan can come with a learning curve—that's normal. As with all lifestyles, there will be challenges, things to learn (and unlearn), and adjustments to make to get the results you're striving for. The key to success is persistence in being intuitive to ensure you're eating a healthy variety of nutrient-dense foods to fuel your body and active lifestyle.

That Healthy Glow

Making the switch to plant-based whole foods can have many health benefits. The American Heart Association says eating a plant-based diet reduces the risk of diseases such as type 2 diabetes, high blood pressure, heart disease, certain cancers, and high cholesterol.

According to Dr. Michael Greger, plant-based diets can also improve mood, boost productivity, and reduce inflammation.

Removing dairy from your diet, for example, can result in a decrease or removal of acne. The Harvard Nurses' Health Study found a positive association between acne and the intake of milk, pointing the finger at the presence of hormones and bioactive molecules in dairy.

That Low Carbon Footprint

It's undeniable that our actions have an impact on the environment. Although veganism may not be the sole action required, it is by far the greatest solution we can take as individuals to combat climate change, deforestation, ecosystem destruction, and species loss and to help lessen our carbon footprint.

When we leave animal products off our plates, we use 50 percent less carbon dioxide, one-eleventh less oil, one-thirteenth less water, and only one-eighteenth of the land, compared with meat eaters, according to research conducted by Cowspiracy.

The United Nations urges people around the world to shift away from eating meat and dairy to help combat world hunger and climate change, as the demand for animal products is having devastating effects on the planet and is not sustainable for the future.

Adopting a vegan lifestyle is a direct action for a more sustainable and compassionate future.

That High-Energy Goodness

The foods you eat play a vital role in your energy levels. If you feed your body well and consume a wide variety of vegetables, nuts, seeds, fruits, and whole grains, you're fueling yourself right for an active lifestyle. Eat the rainbow!

Plant-based foods are among the easiest to digest, which works to your advantage because your body works faster to convert the foods you consume for energy output, rather than taking longer to digest, as is often the case with meat, which can be slower and more difficult to digest.

Stick to It

Consistency is the key. Don't worry about enjoying some vegan comfort foods or takeout once in a while. As long as you stick to your healthy habits more often than you indulge in junk food, you're on the right track. There are also great meat and cheese alternatives available in grocery stores and restaurants that can satisfy any cravings you may have from time to time.

Veganism isn't a diet, it's a lifestyle. It's less about perfection and more about sticking with it over the long run for the sake of the animals, your health, and the planet. Don't let small setbacks discourage you.

Balance Is Key

One of the most common mistakes people make when going vegan is that they simply don't eat enough. The nutrients we need are split into two categories: macronutrients and micronutrients. Macronutrients are carbohydrates, fats, and proteins. Micronutrients are vitamins and minerals. In general terms, we need larger amounts of macronutrients, which are responsible for supplying our calories and providing our energy, and smaller amounts of micronutrients, which play a critical role in keeping our bodies healthy and aiding the digestion of macronutrients. Keeping note of your macronutrient and micronutrient consumption can help ensure that you have healthy eating habits.

Carbohydrates

Carbohydrates, often called carbs, are responsible for providing our body with glucose, which is converted to energy and supports our physical activity. Carbohydrates are the body's main source of fuel and key for brain, kidney, muscle, and heart function. Carbohydrates consist of three components: fiber, starch, and sugar. Not all carbs are created equal, so it's important to choose the right foods to fuel your active lifestyle.

The difference between simple and complex carbs is how quickly the glucose is absorbed and digested. Simple carbs spike blood glucose levels quickly, resulting in short bursts of energy often followed by a crash. Complex carbs raise glucose blood levels more slowly but for longer, providing you with more sustained, ongoing energy.

You can obtain simple carbohydrates from healthy sources such as fruits and vegetables, which also provide the body with vitamins, minerals, and fiber. However, simple carbs are also found in processed foods and those containing added sugars, such as soda pop, candy, pastries, and French fries. These foods should be avoided.

Complex carbohydrates are commonly referred to as good carbs. It's important to choose quality sources instead of refined or processed options, such as white flour or white rice. Some healthy sources of complex carbohydrates are chickpeas, quinoa, brown rice, kidney beans, black beans, lentils, barley, oats, spelt, potatoes, and buckwheat.

Fats

Often misunderstood, fat plays an important role in providing our bodies what they need to function and maintain good health. Fat is an energy reserve that protects our vital organs and assists in the absorption of fat-soluble vitamins.

Choosing healthy fats means consuming monounsaturated and polyunsaturated food sources, such as avocados, cashews, olives, sunflower seeds, chia seeds, almonds, peanuts, pecans, flaxseed, walnuts, pumpkin seeds, and tofu. Such foods are staples in the plant-based lifestyle.

Omega-3 and omega-6 fatty acids are both polyunsaturated fats. They promote and support joint health, the immune system, and brain function, and they can be anti-inflammatory. Registered dietician Jack Norris notes that we must consume alpha-linolenic (ALA), the short-chain fatty acid found in plant-based foods, because the body can't produce it on its own. The body can produce small amounts of the long-chain fatty acids, EPA and DHA, by converting them from ALA. A few great plant-based sources of these fatty acids are walnuts, flaxseed, hemp, and chia seeds. Supplements are also a convenient option.

Unhealthy fats, such as trans-unsaturated and saturated fats (often referred to as the "bad fats"), should be avoided. Trans fats can increase disease risk and raise your low-density lipoprotein (LDL) cholesterol, putting you at risk of a heart attack. Food sources that contain trans fats include those processed using hydrogenated or partially hydrogenated oil, such as fried foods and packaged pastries, crackers, and chips. Saturated fats aren't as harmful as trans fats, but they do also raise LDL ("bad") cholesterol and can also affect heart health. It's best to avoid them as much as possible. Primary sources of saturated fat are red meat, whole-fat dairy products, butter, and cheese. Those of us who have a plant-based lifestyle already avoid these animal-based products. Even vegans, however, should be aware of their consumption of saturated oils, which are present in some plant-based sources like coconut and palm oils.

Proteins

We touched on protein earlier, and we'll be jumping into more details on a few of the essential amino acids responsible for muscle growth and recovery on page 13. Right now, though, let's explore the many high-quality sources of protein vegans can eat.

Remember, you can obtain every amino acid required by the human body from plants. There is nothing meat has that can't be found in plant-based sources.

Some excellent sources of protein are quinoa, tofu, tempeh, beans, lentils, whole grains, oats, brown rice, green peas, amaranth, seitan, and nuts. Meat alternatives can be a great option for convenience or just a treat, but it's best to avoid consuming too many processed foods on a regular basis. It's healthier to opt for less processed options.

Micronutrients

Vitamins and minerals are micronutrients, and both play vital roles in one's health. Vitamins are either water-soluble or fat-soluble, according to Harvard Medical School.

Water-soluble vitamins are easily flushed out through our urine, which means we must replace them regularly. These vitamins and their plant sources are:

B_1 **(thiamine):** pine nuts, sunflower seeds, tahini, watermelon, whole grains

B_2 **(riboflavin):** almonds, avocados, mushrooms, soybeans

B_3 **(niacin):** barley, peanuts, potatoes, spirulina, tomatoes, wild rice

B_6 **(pyridoxine):** almonds, bananas, chickpeas, hemp seeds, kale, soy, watermelon

B$_7$ (biotin): almonds, carrots, chia, oats, sweet potatoes

B$_9$ (folate): artichokes, beans, broccoli, celery, lentils, mangos, oranges, spinach, walnuts

B$_{12}$ (cobalamin): fortified nutritional yeast, fortified plant-based milks (almond, coconut, oat, soy, etc.), or a supplement

Vitamin C: broccoli, Brussels sprouts, grapefruit, kiwi, leafy greens, lemons, oranges, peppers

Fat-soluble vitamins are best absorbed when consumed with a source of fat. They are not lost as easily as water-soluble vitamins, as they accumulate in the body and are not typically needed daily. These vitamins and their plant sources are:

Vitamin A: cantaloupe, carrots, collards, kale, spinach, sweet potatoes

Vitamin D: natural sunshine, fortified plant-based milks (almond, coconut, oat, soy, etc.), or a supplement (D$_2$ is derived from plant sources, whereas D$_3$ is found in animal sources, but there are vegan D$_3$ supplements available)

Vitamin E: almonds, avocados, hazelnuts, leafy greens, sunflower seeds

Vitamin K: cabbage, leafy greens, pumpkin, soybeans

Minerals are also necessary for health, and we need to consume them on a regular basis. They are critical, especially for athletes who deplete their mineral stores more quickly to meet the demands of high-intensity activity. These minerals and their plant sources are:

Calcium: almond butter, black-eyed peas, blackstrap molasses, bok choy, broccoli, fortified plant-based milks, leafy greens, tofu, white beans

Iodine: iodized salt, pink Himalayan salt, seaweed

Iron: beans, dark leafy greens, lentils, nuts, quinoa, whole grains (make sure to consume with vitamin C–rich foods to help aid the absorption of nonheme, or plant-based, iron)

Magnesium: broccoli, seeds, legumes, spinach, whole wheat

Potassium: apricots, bananas, kidney beans, lima beans, potatoes, prunes, sweet potatoes, white beans

Selenium: Brazil nuts (greatest source), long-grain brown rice, oatmeal, whole wheat bread

Sodium: beets, carrots, celery

Zinc: hemp seeds, lentils, mushrooms, oatmeal, pumpkin seeds, spinach, whole grains, wild rice

Nailing Your Nutritional Needs

Nutrition is a huge factor in performance and recovery. It fuels your training and competition and ensures proper muscle recovery to help push you to the next level. Even if you're not very active, making sure your nutrition is on point for your needs can help boost your energy and focus, allowing you to be more productive. By considering your specific goals, body type, and the type of activities you participate in, you can start to determine your personal nutritional needs to thrive and feel your best.

Energy

The three main nutrients that your body uses for energy are carbohydrates, protein, and fats. Of those, carbohydrates are the most important source. Your body can also use protein and fats for energy when you have have depleted your store of carbs. According to the American College of Sports Medicine, however, fat can't produce energy fast enough to meet the needs of intense physical activity, like carbohydrates can, so eating a low-carb diet can hinder high-intensity performance.

Endurance

If you're an endurance athlete, you need carbs. They are a main fuel source and help maintain sufficient blood glucose levels to optimize your muscle and liver glycogen stores. Nitrate-rich vegetables are also important for endurance because they help muscles use the fuel supply more efficiently, which has a positive impact on going the distance.

The repetitive nature of the activities in endurance sports puts stress on the body. Anti-inflammatory foods, such as turmeric, beets, pineapples, blueberries, garlic, leafy greens, nuts, and seeds, help your body cope with this stress, so be sure to include them in your diet.

Strength

When you tell someone you are vegan, they will probably ask, "Where do you get your protein?" In their defense, many people have been conditioned through biased nutritional education and marketing to think meat equals protein. However, more and more people are finally becoming aware that vegans have a vast selection of protein-rich food options.

The stereotype that we need meat to build strength also stems from a misunderstanding of protein itself. As mentioned earlier, all the essential amino acids we require can be found in plant-based foods, making vegan protein easily obtainable, highly digestible, and nutrient-dense. Excellent sources of protein include quinoa, tempeh, tofu, beans, lentils, whole grains, oats, seitan, and nuts, to name just a few. (See Amazing Aminos on page 13 for more about muscle-building aminos.)

Your Personal Goals

No matter what your goals are and whether you're already vegan or just starting out, this book will equip you with the tools to help you reach your potential by customizing the recipes, meal plans, and nutritional recommendations to meet your personal needs. Be intuitive and pay attention to how your body performs and recovers after eating various foods and food combinations. Take note of how you feel when eating certain amounts of different foods before and after being active. Customize the wealth of information, recipes, and recommended resources in these pages so that this book becomes your personal playbook.

AMAZING AMINOS

Amino acids, the building blocks of protein, are essential for muscle growth, especially leucine, isoleucine, and valine. These three essential amino acids are commonly referred to as branched-chain amino acids (BCAAs) because they help support protein synthesis. They play a crucial role in the body's ability to build and maintain muscle, as well as aid recovery. Many vegans and meat-eating athletes reach for BCAAs supplements, but there are plant-based food sources of these key amino acids. It's also important to note that these three amino acids can function as fuel for muscles, so your body will diminish its supplies, making it that much more important to replenish them through the foods you eat. Athletes and those involved in intensive training need more of these BCAAs than sedentary people.

Leucine helps regulate blood sugar levels. It also promotes the growth and recovery of muscle and bone tissue. Leucine can also help minimize the muscle protein breakdown caused by an injury. Sources include chia seeds, firm tofu, flaxseed, hemp seeds, navy beans, and pumpkin seeds.

Isoleucine helps with increased endurance, muscle tissue recovery and repair, blood glucose regulation, and hemoglobin production. Sources include firm tofu, kamut, lentils, podded peas, and pumpkin seeds.

Valine maintains muscle and prevents it from breaking down. It's important for cognitive functions and your nervous system. Sources include firm tofu, navy beans, oatmeal, podded peas, and pumpkin seeds.

How to Determine Your Unique Nutritional Needs

Over the past decade, countless people have asked me for help figuring out their personal caloric and macronutrient needs. Many find it helpful to track their macros and caloric intake, especially when just starting the vegan lifestyle or when they have a specific goal in mind.

Tracking your calories or macros can be effective, but I strongly urge you to be intuitive, as well. For example, if you are still hungry, please don't deprive yourself of a healthy meal or snack simply because you've already hit your "set" caloric or macro goals for the day. It's very important to make sure you give your body the nutrition it requires, especially as an athlete, and understand that any targets you set should be general guidelines. Be open to adjusting these targets as needed.

Fat-Free Mass

Fat-free mass (FFM), sometimes referred to as lean body mass, is everything in your body except fat, including your bones, organs, muscles, and water.

FFM is mainly a reference to your muscle mass. Muscles keep our bodies in motion and burn more calories than fat, so having a good FFM will help your body excel in physical activity and help maintain health.

To determine your FFM, you need to know your body fat percentage. You can use the following formula to calculate your FFM.

weight [kg] × (1 − (body fat [%] / 100)) = FFM [kg]

For example, if you weigh 75 kilograms and have 12 percent body fat, your FFM would be 66 kilograms.

75 × (1 − (12 / 100)) = 66 kg FFM

Note: To figure out your weight in kilograms, the conversion is 1 pound = 0.45359237 kilograms. So, the calculation is: your weight in pounds × 0.45359237 = your weight in kilograms.

Basal Metabolic Rate

Your basal metabolic rate (BMR) is the number of calories your body needs while resting. Knowing your BMR can help you reach your goals by helping you figure out how many calories you need to consume and how many you need to burn.

The Revised Harris Benedict Equations for BMR are as follows:

MEN

88.362 + (13.397 × weight in kilograms)
+ (4.799 × height in centimeters) − (5.677 × age in years) = BMR

WOMEN

447.593 + (9.247 × weight in kilograms)
+ (3.098 × height in centimeters) − (4.330 × age in years) = BMR

For example, a 35-year-old male who weighs 75 kilograms and is 183 centimeters in height would have a BMR of 1,772.65.

88.362 + (13.397 × 75) + (4.799 × 183) − (5.677 × 35) = 1,772.66 BMR

Total Daily Energy Expenditure

Once you've calculated your BMR, you can determine your total daily energy expenditure (TDEE), which is the total number of calories you burn in a day.

Your TDEE looks at your daily activities and includes the amount of energy your body requires to digest and process the food you eat. Additionally, your TDEE includes your nonexercise activity thermogenesis (NEAT), which is the energy you spend during the day doing nonexercise activities, such as walking, climbing stairs at work or school, and working.

There are five formulas to determine this score based on your lifestyle:

1. **Little/no exercise: BMR × 1.2 = TDEE**

2. **Light exercise: BMR × 1.375 = TDEE**

3. **Moderate exercise (3 to 5 days per week): BMR × 1.55 = TDEE**

4. **Very active (6 to 7 days per week): BMR × 1.725 = TDEE**

5. **Extra active (very active plus a physical job): BMR × 1.9 = TDEE**

For example: if your BMR is 1,772.65 and you do moderate exercise 3 to 5 days per week, your TDEE would be 1,772.65 × 1.55 = 2,747.61

Your TDEE provides a rough estimate of how many calories you burn in a day and should be used as a general guide. Adjust your caloric intake as needed.

Daily Caloric Needs and Allowance

You can use your TDEE to adjust the number of calories you consume depending on your needs and goals. You will need to increase or decrease your caloric intake depending on whether you are looking to lose, maintain, or gain weight. Use the formulas provided to help determine your personalized needs, but be intuitive and flexible regarding your individual body, and adjust your targets accordingly.

According to the US Department of Health, the estimated caloric need per day for adult women is 1,600 to 2,400, and for adult men, it is 2,000 to 3,000 per day. For example, the average daily caloric needs of an active male age 31 to 35 is 3,000 calories and for an active woman age 31 to 35 is 2,200 calories.

Consuming insufficient calories can put you at risk for missing essential nutrients, which can affect your health and your ability to participate in demanding athletic activities.

Macronutrient Needs (Protein, Fats, Carbs)

Protein is an essential macronutrient, and the National Academies' Institute of Medicine recommends that adults should aim to get about 0.8 grams of protein per kilogram of body weight. Your protein intake should range from 10 percent to 35 percent of your daily calories.

Athletes, however, need to consume more protein than the average sedentary person. Endurance athletes require 1.2 to 1.4 grams per kilogram of body weight, and bodybuilders and athletes involved in strength training require 1.6 to 2.2 grams per kilogram of body weight.

Fat is also essential for health, so even if you prefer eating a low-fat diet, it's vital that you don't omit fats altogether. Get your fats from quality sources such as avocados, nuts, and seeds. Studies recommend that 20 to 35 percent of the daily calories of an average adult should come from fat. One gram of fat has 9 calories, so that translates to 44 to 77 grams of fat per day based on 2,000 calories per day.

Carbs are a key player in health and athletics, and the average adult should get 45 to 65 percent of their daily calories from carbohydrates. One gram of carbs has about 4 calories, which translates to 225 to 325 grams of carbs per day based on an intake of 2,000 calories per day.

Quick tip! Having a carbohydrate-packed snack or meal within 30 minutes after training gets your body started on restoring glycogen. Consuming meals high in carbs within six hours of training helps that restoration continue, as stated by the United States Anti-Doping Agency.

To sum it all up, the general recommended macronutrient ratio for an average adult is as follows:

Protein: 10% to 35%

Fat: 20% to 35%

Carbohydrates: 45% to 65%

Remember, these ratios are based on an average adult and are shown here for general guidance. You will need to adjust your ratios and caloric intake based on your individual needs, goals, physical activity, and preferences.

Online calculators for FFM, body mass index, BMR, TDEE, macros, and calories, are available at www.MeatFreeAthlete.com/calculators.

CHEAT DAYS

Cheat days—or flex days, as you may prefer to call them—are when you eat foods that aren't necessarily on your meal plan or suited to help you meet your personal goals. I avoid using the term "cheat" because people may associate guilt with what they eat or develop a negative relationship with particular foods.

There are vegan versions of practically all your favorite snacks and fast foods, from ice cream to burgers to pizza, so you have lots of great options to choose from without reaching for the nonvegan counterparts.

It's all about balance. Having a flex day or meal in the vegan lifestyle is completely fine, and there's nothing wrong with allowing yourself to stray occasionally from your regular healthier routine. In fact, I encourage you to do so. Feeling restricted or associating shame with certain foods or meals may cause you to develop an unhealthy relationship with food. Thriving as a vegan athlete isn't solely about your athletic performance or aesthetics; it's also about your mental health and overall well-being.

How to Use This Book Like a Champ

This book has been created to equip you with more than 100 plant-powered recipes, a baseline understanding of essential nutrients, and easy-to-follow action items, meal plans, and formulas to help you calculate your personalized needs so you can start incorporating them into your daily routine today.

Be Prepared

Those who fail to prepare should prepare to fail. Achieving your goals requires dedication to planning, preparation, and perseverance. Keeping your kitchen well-stocked and functional will make your journey much easier and set you up for success. The next chapter provides shopping tips and best practices for meal prep.

The Plans

Coming up, I provide three easy-to-follow meal plans, based on various goals: energy, endurance, and strength. These plans include macro and calorie totals for the week and are meant as best-practice general guidelines. Keep in mind that everyone has different caloric and macro requirements based on their weight and activity level. You will be able to customize the meal plans to best suit your nutritional needs and goals. Please note that this book and its information should be used as a guideline and supplement, not as a replacement for advice from your personal physician. If you have any health concerns, make sure to speak with your doctor before getting started.

Recipes

I've packed this cookbook with 101 delicious, no-fuss vegan recipes and focused on providing easy, nutrient-dense meals that will help you maximize your results. There are no weird or hard-to-find ingredients. I keep it simple and affordable, while veganizing many of your favorite dishes.

These recipes emphasize using a variety of healthy, plant-based whole foods, leaving out processed and store-bought meat substitutes, but I've included some comfort foods, too. You'll find some canned and frozen foods as ingredient options for the sake of ease, time-saving, and cost-efficiency.

Meat alternatives are useful for those newly transitioning to the vegan lifestyle, or for occasional convenience. It's important, especially as athletes, to focus on whole foods most of the time, for better digestion and to ensure that your nutrient intake is keeping up with your active lifestyle.

The recipes have labels (Energy Boost, Strength Builder, Pre-Game, Recovery, and Grab and Go) so you can quickly find exactly what you're looking for to meet your nutritional or performance needs and personal preferences.

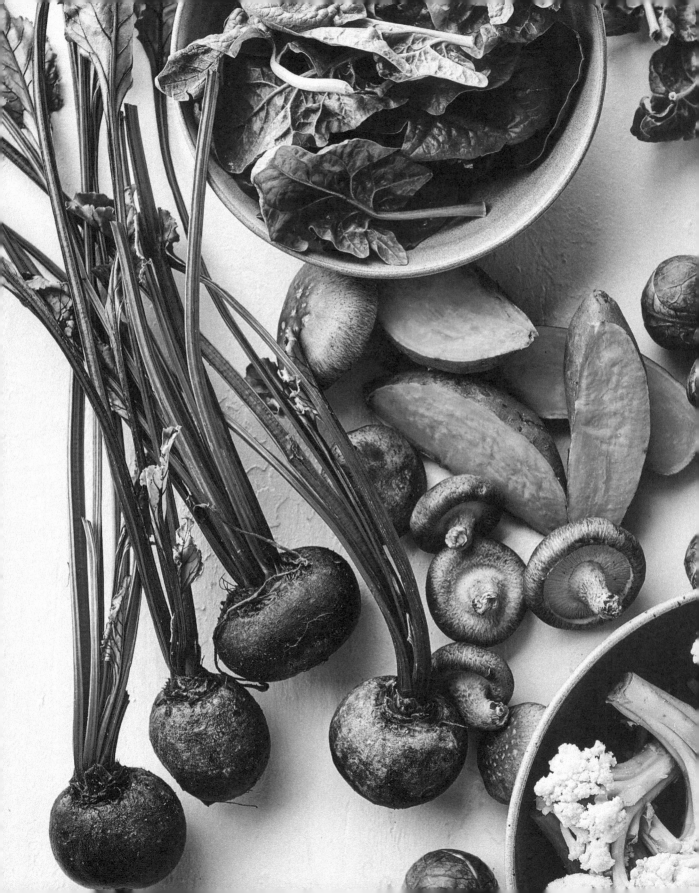

CHAPTER 2

Get Your Pantry Performance-Ready

When I went vegan, I discovered a new appreciation for the food I eat and where it comes from. I started cooking more of my own meals, learned how to veganize my favorite dishes, and discovered healthy, plant-based alternatives to more traditional foods. I quickly realized my kitchen needed a makeover. I made it a priority to stock up on the necessary foods and ingredients and to acquire the right tools to make it easy to prepare healthy meals.

Shop Like a Pro

Part of a successful game plan includes having a strategy for grocery shopping. The way you shop is an important part of your meal prep. Here are some key tips.

Check Before You Buy

Check your refrigerator and pantry before going shopping to avoid buying items you already have.

Have a Weekly Meal Plan

Plan meals for the week ahead that include similar ingredients so you can use up what you buy. Select meals based on the activities planned that week to help you stay on track with your athletic goals, nutritional needs, and budget.

Make a List

After checking your kitchen and preparing your meal plan, make a list of exactly what you need. This will help ensure you don't forget anything. You can also save money by buying only what's on your prepared list and avoiding unplanned purchases.

Eat Before You Shop

Shopping on an empty stomach encourages impulse buys. If you are between meals, grab a quick snack before heading out to keep you focused on buying only the items you intended to get on your list.

Buy in Bulk

Buying in bulk is an excellent way to save money on staples such as beans, lentils, grains, nuts, seeds, spices, and herbs. It's also an eco-friendly option when you can reuse your own containers and bags.

Buy It Frozen

Fresh fruits and vegetables can be expensive and often go bad before you use them. Avoid waste and save money by purchasing frozen fruits and vegetables. These foods are frozen immediately after harvest and retain as many or even more nutrients than their fresh counterparts.

Read Labels

Reading food labels is a good habit. Not all vegan products will be labeled as such, so look through the ingredient list to spot any animal-based food sources. Also check out the macros (fat, carbs, protein) on the nutrition facts label, and keep an eye out for processed sugar.

COOKING WITHOUT OILS

The recipes in this book are made without oil, but cooking without added oils does not mean we'll be avoiding dietary fat, which is essential for health and necessary for absorbing fat-soluble nutrients.

Why omit oil as a primary source of healthy fat? Oil is highly processed, which strips the whole food—whether olives, avocados, or coconuts—of its nutrients. The result is a 100 percent fat, nutrient-poor, and calorically dense product.

According to Dr. Caldwell B. Esselstyn in a paper in the *International Journal of Disease Reversal and Prevention*, both the monounsaturated and saturated fats contained in oils are harmful to the endothelium, the innermost lining of the artery. This damage is the gateway to vascular disease. Additionally, endothelial function declines for several hours after oil consumption, decreasing and restricting blood flow. This should be a cause for concern for anyone, especially those participating in high-intensity activity.

Dr. Esselstyn studied seriously ill coronary artery disease patients who were given a whole food, plant-based nutrition plan that excluded all oils. He reported on this study at 5 years, 12 years, 16 years, and 20 years in peer-reviewed scientific journals, as discussed in his book, *Prevent and Reverse Heart Disease*. The results showed a huge drop in cholesterol levels, the disappearance of angina, and weight loss. In some patients, X-rays demonstrated disease reversal, proving that previously blocked arteries were no longer present.

It makes no difference if the oil is extra-virgin olive oil, coconut oil, corn oil, or canola oil. They all have the same adverse effect on heart health. Even though these oils are plant-based, you should avoid or limit them. The eating style proposed in this book is not about perfection, though, so if you do consume oil sporadically, don't sweat it. Just get back on track.

When you follow the meal plans and recipes in this book, you'll be consuming all your essential fats straight from nutrient-dense sources, such as avocados, nuts, seeds, hemp seeds, olives, coconuts, and flaxseed. Cooking without oil takes a little practice at first, but you will quickly get the hang of it.

Quality Equipment

Having the right tools on hand will help make meal preparation easy. Let's take a look at some staple items you need in your vegan kitchen.

Equipment

Citrus Press

There are many citrus presses out there, manual and electric. Manual presses cost less and still do a great job, so there's no need to spend a lot. Using a citrus press will make it easier to get more juice while keeping out the seeds.

Cutting Boards

A high-quality cutting board is important for safety and for keeping your knives sharp. Get a cutting board that grips to the counter well and doesn't slip around, both to decrease the risk of cutting yourself and to protect your countertop from cut marks.

Knives

You're going to be doing a lot of cutting, dicing, and mincing. A good set of sharp knives will make all this prep work easier and save you time. It is also much safer to use a sharp knife because you can cut with more precision and less pressure. Invest in a decent set of knives and keep them sharpened.

Parchment Paper

This is a staple item in the kitchen, especially when cooking without oil. Use parchment paper to line baking sheets and casserole dishes; it successfully prevents foods from sticking to cookware. You can reuse it, and compost when you're finished with it.

Pots and Pans

When you're cooking at home on a regular basis, you need a good set of pots and pans, inclucing saucepans, frying pans, skillets, and stockpots. Invest in quality nonstick cookware; it is a staple for oil-free cooking and will last a long time if you take good care of it. Avoid using metal utensils and wash the pans by hand so the coating doesn't scratch off.

Make sure your pots and pans are free of perfluorooctanoic acid (PFOA). This synthetic chemical can contaminate the water, soil, and air during the manu-facturing process. Many nonstick brands offer PFOA-free options.

Silicone Cookware

Silicone cookware is great for oil-free baking. These nonstick items come in many shapes, from baking sheet liners to cupcake molds and muffin cups. They are made from food-grade silicone and are free of bisphenol A (BPA), an indus-trial chemical found in many food containers. They are also reusable, durable, oven-safe up to 480°F, flexible, and easy to clean.

Appliances

Air Fryer

Air fryers make fried foods without the oil. Many air fryers recommend using a little oil, but I've never used oil and I get great results. I really enjoy my air fryer; the possibilities are endless. Check out Air-Fried Spring Rolls (page 76) for a healthier version of this traditionally deep-fried food.

Food Processor

A food processor is an essential piece of equipment for chopping, blending, kneading, or mixing. The blades do the heavy work and make it easier and faster to prepare food. There is no need to buy an expensive food processor; the budget-friendly brands work well.

Slow Cooker

A slow cooker allows you to prepare a meal by putting all your ingredients into the pot at once, covering them with the lid, and cooking, unattended, at a low temperature over several hours. It's a great option when you want to come home to a hot meal.

Vegetable Steamer

Steaming is a quick and healthy way to cook vegetables, and a vegetable steamer basket is the easiest method. Insert the basket into a pot or pan that has water in the bottom, cover the pot with a lid, and heat it on the stovetop.

Storage

Reusable Containers

Good-quality food storage containers are essential for meal prep and storing leftovers. I recommend glass containers that are safe for use in the refrigerator, freezer, oven, microwave, and dishwasher. Along with being versatile, glass containers are also more environmentally friendly than plastic. If you already have plastic containers, use what you have available, and when they become worn down, remember to recycle them.

Mason jars are great for storing soups, sauces, and leftovers. They come in a variety of sizes and are easy to find in stores. Some pasta sauces, jams, and soups come in Mason jars, which you can clean out and reuse.

The Power of Meal Prep

Meal prep is different from meal planning. Meal prep is when you prepare your meals ahead of time.

The goal of meal prep is to make it easier to stay on track with your goals. I recommend doing meal prep twice a week, on Sunday and either Wednesday or

Thursday, but you can prepare all your meals on the weekend or on your days off to fit your schedule. You'll save money and eat more healthfully if you avoid dining out at restaurants or buying convenience foods.

Committing to focusing on your health and mental well-being is a form of self-care. Be your own biggest fan and become dedicated to building your best self. You are your only true competition, so be your biggest supporter, too!

Keep Your Nutritional Goals in Mind

When you are meal planning, keep your athletic and nutritional goals top of mind. Are you trying to maintain, gain, or lose weight? Are you looking to gain muscle? The meals you prepare should be geared toward helping you achieve that.

By planning and preparing your meals in advance, you can focus on portion size and your daily caloric needs. This also will help you keep track of your macros and overall nutritional intake. Your target needs will likely shift and change over time. Preparing your meals each week allows you to pivot and adjust when necessary.

Reuse Ingredients for Efficiency

Preparing your meals ahead of time allows you to strategically make dishes that use many of the same ingredients. This will help you save time and money and cut back on tossing out unused groceries. It is much easier to prepare meals with shared ingredients.

Start simple. Once you get comfortable with the process, you can start to branch out from the meal plans provided and adapt them to meet your specific needs. This way of preparing meals will soon become second nature.

Take It Easy

Meal prep is a tool to help you reach your goals and save time and money. It takes practice and intuition, but the more you do it, the better you'll get and the easier it will become. Take your time, learn, and enjoy the process.

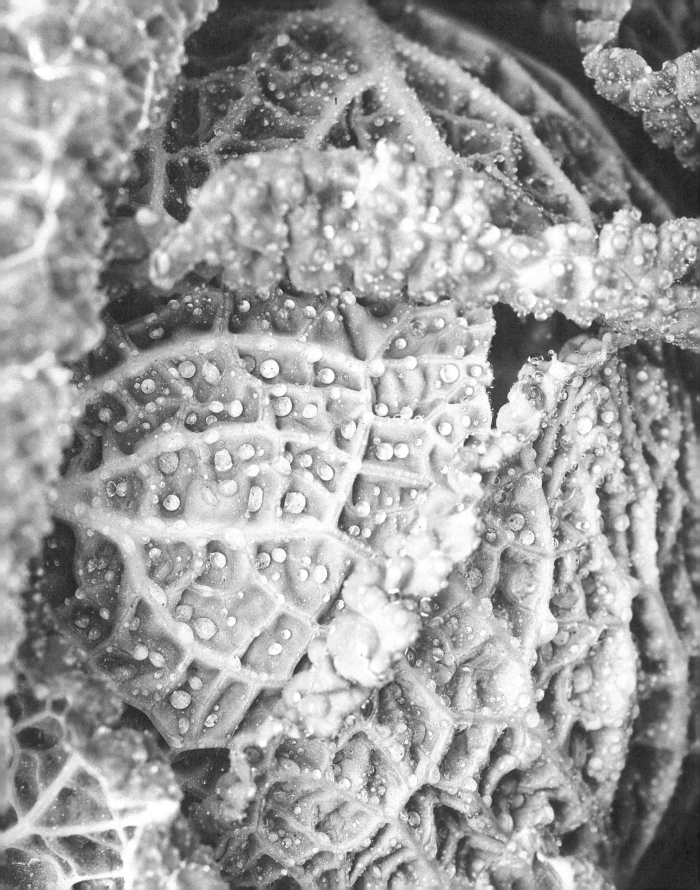

CHAPTER 3

Eat for the Gold

This chapter provides three seven-day meal plans specifically designed to suit your different athletic endeavors: strength, endurance, and energy. Each plan includes meals, snacks, and pre-workout and post-workout suggestions to help maximize your performance and recovery.

I've included shopping lists for each plan, so you know exactly what you need for the week. There are a lot of easy recipes, and convenient grab-and-go options. Each weekly plan has been developed to make meal prep easier and avoid food waste.

Each meal plan has suggestions based on general needs. You will need to use the tools provided in this book, such as the TDEE formula (page 15), to gain a greater understanding of your personal nutritional needs.

Adjust these meal plans based on your individual caloric needs, the intensity of your workouts, and your metabolism, goals, and preferences.

If you're looking to gain more mass, try adding 100 to 200 calories per day to your TDEE for a week. If you're looking to lose, try removing those calories. Monitor your progress weekly (or monthly) and adjust accordingly.

Energy Plan

When we eat foods our body thrives on, we can optimize our performance, improve our overall health, and benefit from sustained energy. All athletes should pay close attention to their energy levels throughout the day to get a clear picture of what works best for them. There isn't a one-size-fits-all solution, so it's important to take note of how you feel when you eat certain foods and at which times of the day you consume them. From there, you can adjust as needed, depending on the demands of your schedule and athletic activities.

I'm not completely against caffeine, but I recommend avoiding it as much as possible in order to get a true picture of whether you're getting energy from the foods you are eating or from caffeine. The natural energy you gain from a whole food, plant-based lifestyle can also help improve your focus, motivation, and mood.

Prioritize eating more fiber and foods with high water content, such as cucumbers, tomatoes, spinach, mushrooms, watermelon, oranges, pineapples, celery, beans, lentils, and bananas.

Shopping List

Canned and Bottled Items

Applesauce, unsweetened, 1 (24-ounce) jar

Beans, black, 1 (19-ounce) can

Broth, vegetable, 1 (14.5-ounce) can

Chickpeas, 1 (19-ounce) can

Pantry

Almonds, whole, 1 (3.5-ounce) bag

Baking powder

Baking soda

Bread, whole wheat, 1 (24-ounce) loaf

Cashews, raw, 8 ounces

Cranberries, dried, 1 (6-ounce) bag

Flaxseed, ground

Flour, chickpea

Flour, whole wheat

Maple syrup

Mustard, Dijon

Mustard, yellow

Nutritional yeast, B_{12}-fortified

Oats, rolled

Oats, steel-cut

Pasta, chickpea-based

Quinoa

Rice, brown

Rice, wild

Seeds, ground chia

Seeds, hulled hemp

Spirulina

Tahini

TVP (textured vegetable protein), dried

Vanilla extract

Vinegar, apple cider

Vinegar, balsamic

Vital wheat gluten

Fresh Produce

Apples, Granny Smith (12)

Avocados (5)

Bananas (6)

Bell peppers, red (3)

Bok choy (1 bunch)

Celery (1 bunch)

Cucumbers (3)

Dates, Medjool (8 ounces)

Garlic (1 head)

Ginger (1 root)

Kale (13 cups)

Lemons (4)

Mushrooms (8 ounces)

Mushrooms, cremini (½ cup)

Onion, red (1)

Onions, yellow (2)

Oranges (3)

Parsley (1 bunch)

Potatoes, sweet (2)

Scallions (1 bunch)

Spinach (18 cups)

Tomatoes (6)

Tomatoes, cherry (1 pint)

Zucchini (1)

Frozen Produce

Beets, 2 (10-ounce) bags

Blueberries, 2 (16-ounce) bags

Broccoli florets, 1 (16-ounce) bag

Cherries, 1 (16-ounce) bag

Edamame, shelled, 3 (10-ounce) bags

Pineapple, 4 (16-ounce) bags

Raspberries, 1 (16-ounce) bag

Strawberries, 1 (16-ounce) bag

Spices

Basil, dried

Cinnamon, ground

Garlic powder

Italian seasoning

Onion powder

Oregano, dried

Pepper, black

Salt, pink Himalayan

Turmeric

Vegan chick'n bouillon

Vegan poultry seasoning

Other

Plant-based milk, unsweetened (1 gallon)

Tofu, firm, 3 (350-gram) blocks

Equipment List

Air fryer (or oven)

Blender

Citrus press

Cutting board

Food processor

Knives

Mason jars with lids

Measuring cups and spoons

Mixing bowls

Muffin pan

Nonstick baking sheet

Nonstick skillets and pots

Parchment paper or silicone sheet

Storage containers, reusable

Vegetable steamer

Meal Plan

	MONDAY	TUESDAY	WEDNESDAY	THURSDAY
BREAKFAST	Apple-Cinnamon Quinoa (page 64)	Apple-Cinnamon Quinoa	Tofu Scramble (page 71)	Tofu Scramble
PRE-WORKOUT	Very Berry Antioxidant Smoothie (page 62)	Very Berry Antioxidant Smoothie	Very Berry Antioxidant Smoothie	Apple-Cinnamon Quinoa
POST-WORKOUT	Green Power Smoothie (page 60) *Optional: add 2 tablespoons pea protein powder for 30 grams of additional protein*	Green Power Smoothie *Optional: add 2 tablespoons pea protein powder for 30 grams of additional protein*	Beet Blast Smoothie (page 59) *Optional: add 2 tablespoons pea protein powder for 30 grams of additional protein*	Green Power Smoothie *Optional: add 2 tablespoons pea protein powder for 30 grams of additional protein*
LUNCH	Alkaline Protein Power Salad (page 79) (½ portion)	Alkaline Protein Power Salad (½ portion)	Chickpea Salad Sandwich (page 92)	Chickpea Salad Sandwich
SNACK	Cranberry-Almond Muffin (page 167)	1 cup steamed shelled edamame with 1 tablespoon B_{12}-fortified nutritional yeast	Cranberry-Almond Muffin	1 cup steamed shelled edamame with 1 tablespoon B_{12}-fortified nutritional yeast
DINNER	Turmeric Italian Tofu and Rice (page 150) with side salad (spinach, tomato, cucumber, green onion, balsamic vinegar)	Turmeric Italian Tofu and Rice with side salad (spinach, tomato, cucumber, green onion, balsamic vinegar)	Spaghetti & Meat-Free Meatballs (page 153) with side salad (spinach, tomato, cucumber, green onion, balsamic vinegar)	Spaghetti & Meat-Free Meatballs with side salad (spinach, tomato, cucumber, green onion, balsamic vinegar)

(continued)

Meal Plan (continued)

		FRIDAY	SATURDAY	SUNDAY
BREAKFAST		¼ cup dry steel-cut oats with 1 orange and 1 banana	Chickpea Omelet (page 68)	Chickpea Omelet
PRE-WORKOUT		Apple-Cinnamon Quinoa	¼ cup dry steel-cut oats with 1 orange and 1 banana	¼ cup dry steel-cut oats with 1 orange and 1 banana
POST-WORKOUT		Green Power Smoothie *Optional: add 2 tablespoons pea protein powder for 30 grams of additional protein*	Beet Blast Smoothie *Optional: add 2 tablespoons pea protein powder for 30 grams of additional protein*	Green Power Smoothie *Optional: add 2 tablespoons pea protein powder for 30 grams of additional protein*
LUNCH		½ cup Turmeric Hummus (page 184) with ½ cucumber, 5 cherry tomatoes, 1 celery stalk	Spaghetti & Meat-Free Meatballs	Spaghetti & Meat-Free Meatballs
SNACK		Cranberry-Almond Muffin	½ cup Turmeric Hummus with ½ cucumber, 5 cherry tomatoes, 1 celery stalk	1 cup steamed shelled edamame with 1 tablespoon B_{12}-fortified nutritional yeast
DINNER		Alkaline Protein Power Salad	Air-Fried Chicken-Style Seitan (page 127) with baked sweet potato, 1 cup steamed broccoli, and 1 cup steamed bok choy	Air-Fried Chicken-Style Seitan with baked sweet potato, 1 cup steamed broccoli, and 1 cup steamed bok choy

Total Macros and Calories for the Week:

Calories: 15,796

Protein: 841 grams

Carbs: 2,462 grams

Fat: 384 grams

Putting the optional scoop of vegan protein powder in your post-workout smoothie could add up to 30 grams of protein and about 170 calories per day.

Step-by-Step Prep

PREP DAY #1—SUNDAY

Prepare the Very Berry Antioxidant Smoothie (page 62), Beet Blast Smoothie (page 59), and Green Power Smoothie (page 60) today and store them in your freezer. Remember, they will take a little bit of time to thaw before you can drink them, so remove them from the freezer ahead of time. Mason jars are great for storing smoothies.

The Apple-Cinnamon Quinoa (page 64) recipe makes 1 serving. Because this meal plan calls for the recipe 4 times, quadruple the recipe. Put the 4 servings into individual reusable containers and store them in the refrigerator.

Tofu Scramble (page 71) makes 2 servings. It is in the meal plan twice, so you can store it in a single container (to save space in your refrigerator), or divide it between 2 containers after it cools.

Alkaline Protein Power Salad (page 79) is for lunch on Monday and Tuesday and for dinner on Friday. This salad includes quinoa and wild rice, so it isn't your average salad. I suggest preparing the lunches today and making the Friday dinner serving on your Thursday prep day. If you choose to prep it all at once, double the recipe. The dinner salad is the full 2 servings, while each lunch is a ½ serving.

Cranberry-Almond Muffins (page 167) are easy to make and store well in a container at room temperature. Store leftovers in the freezer for another time.

Turmeric Italian Tofu and Rice (page 150) consists of sautéing vegetables with tofu and cooking rice. You eat this twice: for dinner on Monday and Tuesday. You will need 2 containers to store it in the refrigerator. This meal has a side salad you can also prepare in advance. Store it in a separate container, with the balsamic dressing kept separate from the salad, until ready to eat.

Chickpea Salad Sandwich (page 92) is a 2-serving recipe. This is your lunch for Wednesday and Thursday. Store it in the refrigerator. Place on the bread when ready to eat.

Steam the edamame for 5 to 7 minutes once the water starts to boil, then store it in the refrigerator. You will be eating 3 cups of edamame this week, and you can eat it warm or cold.

Turmeric Hummus (page 184) is a 2-serving recipe. Transfer the prepared hummus to 2 containers and store in the refrigerator. Then cut up your veggies and refrigerate them, as well.

Spaghetti & Meat-Free Meatballs (page 153) will require a food processor (or blender), and you will need to bake the "meatballs" for 20 to 25 minutes at 350°F. You will cook 8 ounces of chickpea-based pasta until tender. Divide it into 4 equal portions. This is for 4 servings, used for 2 dinners and 2 lunches.

PREP DAY #2—THURSDAY

Steel-cut oats will last in the refrigerator for up to 5 days, getting softer as they sit. To prepare your 3 servings, combine ¾ cup of steel oats with 2¼ cups of water, bring to a boil, and simmer until the oats are soft. Divide the batch into 3 equal portions and store them in containers in the refrigerator. Grab the oranges and bananas when ready to eat.

Chickpea Omelet (page 68) is for breakfast on Saturday and Sunday. Make these omelets separately and store in containers in the refrigerator.

Air-Fried Chicken-Style Seitan (page 127) is made in an air fryer, but you can also bake it on a baking sheet lined with parchment paper or a on silicone sheet in an oven preheated to 350°F if you don't have an air fryer. You will also bake 2 sweet potatoes, steaming 2 cups of broccoli, and 2 cups of bok choy. Store Saturday's and Sunday's dinners separately in 2 containers in the refrigerator.

Endurance Plan

Endurance athletes participate in a variety of sports, including long-distance running, swimming, cycling, soccer, martial arts, and basketball, to name just a few. This endurance plan focuses on developing the circulatory and respiratory systems to provide your muscles with the necessary energy to support prolonged activity.

Aim to consume a variety of nutrient-dense foods and complex carbohydrates while avoiding processed products. Focus on beans, whole grains, oats, lentils, quinoa, sweet potatoes, beets, and leafy greens. Vegetables are key players because they are nitrate-rich and loaded with antioxidants, which can improve blood flow and help deliver oxygen and other nutrients to muscles. Vegetables are also anti-inflammatory, which can be especially important for endurance athletes who put their bodies under a lot of stress with repetitive movements for long periods. Vegetables also get our bodies out of an acidic state after activity. Make vegetables a priority; eat a wide variety and in plentiful amounts. I steam up a big batch of vegetables with most of my dinners, regardless of what the meal is. If you're not a big fan of veggies, start out by eating a lot of the ones you do like. Then begin incorporating new vegetables into the mix. Over time you will discover more vegetables that you enjoy.

Shopping List

Canned and Bottled Items

Beans, black, 1 (19-ounce) can

Beans, pinto, 1 (19-ounce) can

Beans, red kidney, 1 (19-ounce) can

Beans, white kidney, 1 (19-ounce) can

Chickpeas, 1 (19-ounce) can

Pasta sauce, red, vegan, 1 (24-ounce) jar

Tomatoes, diced, 2 (28-ounce) cans

Pantry

Bread, Ezekiel, 1 (24-ounce) loaf

Bread, whole wheat,
1 (24-ounce) loaf

Cashews, raw, 20 ounces

Flaxseed, ground

Flour, whole wheat

Maple syrup

Mustard, Dijon

Nut butter

Nutritional yeast, B_{12}-fortified

Oats, rolled

Oats, steel-cut

Pasta, chickpea-based

Quinoa

Rice, wild

Seeds, hulled hemp

Spirulina

Tempeh, bacon-flavored

Tortillas, whole wheat

Vanilla extract

Vegan dark chocolate chips

Vinegar, apple cider

Vinegar, balsamic

Vital wheat gluten

Fresh Produce

Apples, Granny Smith (7)

Avocados (5)

Bananas (7)

Bell peppers, red (3)

Cherries (16 ounces)

Cucumbers (2)

Garlic (1 head)

Ginger (1 root)

Kale (8 cups)

Lemons (2)

Lettuce, romaine (1 head)

Mushrooms (5 cups)

Onion, red (1)

Onions, yellow (3)

Potatoes, yellow (2)

Scallions (1 bunch)

Spinach (15 cups)

Strawberries (8 ounces)

Tomatoes (6)

Frozen Produce

Beets, 3 (10-ounce) bags

Blueberries, 2 (16-ounce) bags

Broccoli florets, 2 (16-ounce) bags

Cherries, 1 (16-ounce) bag

Coconut, grated, 1 (12-ounce) bag

Corn, 1 (16-ounce) bag

Edamame, shelled, 3 (10-ounce) bags

Peas, green, 1 (16-ounce) bag

Pineapple, 8 (16-ounce) bags

Spices

Basil, dried

Cayenne pepper

Chili powder

Cinnamon, ground

Cumin, ground

Garlic powder

Onion powder

Oregano, dried

Pepper, black

Salt, pink Himalayan

Turmeric

Vegan chick'n bouillon

Vegan poultry seasoning

Other

Coconut milk, unsweetened (not canned), ½ gallon

Plant-based milk, unsweetened, 1 gallon

Tofu, firm, 4 (350-gram) blocks

Equipment List

Air fryer (or oven)

Blender

Citrus press

Cutting board

Food processor

Knives

Mason jars with lids

Measuring cups and spoons

Mixing bowls

Nonstick baking sheet

Nonstick skillets and pots

Parchment paper or silicone sheet

Storage containers, reusable

Vegetable steamer

Meal Plan

	MONDAY	TUESDAY	WEDNESDAY	THURSDAY
BREAKFAST	Cinnamon French Toast (page 69) with ½ cup strawberries	Cinnamon French Toast with ½ cup strawberries	2 slices Ezekiel bread, 2 tablespoons nut butter, and 1 tablespoon hemp seeds	Tofu Scramble (page 71)
PRE-WORKOUT	Beet Blast Smoothie (page 59)	Green Power Smoothie (page 60)	¼ cup dry steel-cut oats with 1 banana and 1 cup cherries	Green Power Smoothie
POST-WORKOUT	Tropical Bliss Smoothie (page 61) *Optional: add 2 tablespoons pea protein powder for 30 grams of additional protein*	Tropical Bliss Smoothie *Optional: add 2 tablespoons pea protein powder for 30 grams of additional protein*	Green Power Smoothie *Optional: add 2 tablespoons pea protein powder for 30 grams of additional protein*	Tropical Bliss Smoothie *Optional: add 2 tablespoons pea protein powder for 30 grams of additional protein*
LUNCH	Alkaline Protein Power Salad (page 79) (½ serving)	Alkaline Protein Power Salad (½ serving)	Ricotta Red Sauce Pasta	5-Bean Chili
SNACK	1 cup steamed shelled edamame with 1 tablespoon B_{12}-fortified nutritional yeast	2 No-Bake Chocolate Chip Bites (page 168)	2 No-Bake Chocolate Chip Bites	1 cup steamed shelled edamame with 1 tablespoon B_{12}-fortified nutritional yeast
DINNER	Ricotta Red Sauce Pasta (page 156) and 2 cups steamed broccoli	5-Bean Chili (page 126) with side salad (spinach, tomato, cucumber, green onion, balsamic vinegar)	Air-Fried Chicken-Style Seitan (page 127), with baked potato and 1 cup steamed green peas	Air-Fried Chicken-Style Seitan, with baked potato and 1 cup steamed green peas

	FRIDAY	SATURDAY	SUNDAY
BREAKFAST	Tofu Scramble	Tofu Scramble	Tofu Scramble
PRE-WORKOUT	Beet Blast Smoothie	Green Power Smoothie	¼ cup dry steel-cut oats with 1 banana and 1 cup cherries
POST-WORKOUT	Tropical Bliss Smoothie *Optional: add 2 tablespoons pea protein powder for 30 grams of additional protein*	Beet Blast Smoothie *Optional: add 2 tablespoons pea protein powder for 30 grams of additional protein*	Tropical Bliss Smoothie *Optional: add 2 tablespoons pea protein powder for 30 grams of additional protein*
LUNCH	5-Bean Chili	5-Bean Chili	Club Wrap
SNACK	1 cup steamed shelled edamame with 1 tablespoon B_{12}-fortified nutritional yeast	2 No-Bake Chocolate Chip Bites	2 No-Bake Chocolate Chip Bites
DINNER	Ricotta Red Sauce Pasta and 2 cups steamed broccoli	Club Wrap (page 93) with side salad (spinach, tomato, cucumber, green onion, balsamic vinegar)	5-Bean Chili with side salad (spinach, tomato, cucumber, green onion, balsamic vinegar)

Total Macros and Calories for the Week:

Calories: 15,526

Protein: 782 grams

Carbs: 2,361 grams

Fat: 437 grams

Putting the optional scoop of vegan protein powder in your post-workout smoothie could add up to 30 grams of protein and about 170 calories per day.

Step-by-Step Prep

PREP DAY #1—SUNDAY

Prepare the Tropical Bliss Smoothie (page 61), Beet Blast Smoothie (page 59), and Green Power Smoothie (page 60) today and store them in your freezer. Remember, they will take a little bit of time to thaw before drinking, so remove them from the freezer ahead of time. Mason jars are great for storing smoothies.

Cinnamon French Toast (page 69) is a 2-serving recipe that can be stored in the same container in the refrigerator for up to 2 days; this is your breakfast on Monday and Tuesday.

Prepare the steel-cut oats for Wednesday's pre-workout fuel (you'll make Sunday's oats during Wednesday's prep session). To make them, combine ¼ cup of steel oats with ¾ cup of water, bring to a boil, and simmer until the oats are soft. Transfer to a container, add the fresh cherries, and store in the refrigerator. Add the banana when you're ready to eat.

Alkaline Protein Power Salad (page 79) will be used for lunch on Monday and Tuesday. This salad includes quinoa and wild rice, which you will prepare today, along with cutting up the veggies and kale. Split the salad into 2 equal portions and store in the refrigerator.

Steam the edamame for 5 to 7 minutes once the water starts to boil, then store in the refrigerator. There are 3 cups of edamame this week, and you can eat it warm or cold.

No-Bake Chocolate Chip Bites (page 168) are quick to throw together and are used as snacks 4 times this week. Store them in a container at room temperature or in the refrigerator. If you will be out of the house at snack time, separate the portions into different containers or reusable baggies and take them with you.

Ricotta Red Sauce Pasta (page 156) requires a food processor (or blender). This is in the meal plan 3 times this week, so you will need 3 containers. Freeze any leftovers to eat another time. You will also prepare 4 cups of steamed broccoli (2 cups each for the dinner on Monday and Friday).

You will need a big pot to cook 5-Bean Chili (page 126). It takes about 45 minutes to cook, so use this time to prepare other items on your list for today. *Tip:* Save the aquafaba (the liquid from the can of chickpeas) and store it in the refrigerator. You can use it on Wednesday to prepare the Mighty Mayo for the Club Wrap.

PREP DAY #2—WEDNESDAY

Air-Fried Chicken-Style Seitan (page 127) is made in an air fryer, but you can also bake it in the oven at 350°F on parchment paper or a silicone sheet if you don't have an air fryer. You will also be baking 2 potatoes and steaming 2 cups of green peas. Store Wednesday's and Thursday's dinners separately in 2 containers in the refrigerator.

Prepare the steel-cut oats for Sunday. To make them, combine ¼ cup of steel oats with ¾ cup of water, bring to a boil, and simmer until the oats are soft. Transfer to a container, add the fresh cherries, and store in the refrigerator. Add the banana when you're ready to eat.

Tofu Scramble (page 71) is a 2-serving recipe, and you are having it 4 times this week. Double the recipe and cook it all at once in a large nonstick skillet. Divide into 4 equal parts, and store in the refrigerator in separate containers.

You can prepare Club Wraps (page 93) in advance by separating the ingredients into containers. Don't put the ingredients in the wrap until you are ready to eat or it will get soggy. Make the side salad for dinner and store in its own container with the balsamic vinegar kept separate.

Strength Plan

For athletes who participate in sports that require power and size, strength is the goal. These sports include football, hockey, rugby, CrossFit, bodybuilding, power-lifting, and weightlifting. It is absolutely possible to build muscle and strength as a vegan. To gradually gain muscle mass, you will need to eat more calories than your daily maintenance requirements, and then use it to power your training. If you don't train enough to match your increased food consumption, you will likely gain weight without the muscle growth or increased strength.

Focus on eating substantial portions of foods such as beans, whole grains, tofu, tempeh, nuts, seeds, and avocados, as well as nitrate-rich leafy greens, which aid in increasing muscle efficiency. If you are not able to consume enough to match your activity and goals, supplementing with a high-quality vegan protein powder can be a convenient way to help hit your targets.

Shopping List

Canned and Bottled Items

Beans, black, 1 (19-ounce) can

Broth, vegetable, 1 (14.5-ounce) can

Chickpeas, 2 (19-ounce) cans

Pantry

Almonds, raw, 6 ounces

Bread, Ezekiel, 1 (24-ounce) loaf

Bread, whole wheat, 1 (24-ounce) loaf

Cashews, 8 ounces

Flour, chickpea

Flour, whole wheat

Jalapeños

Maple syrup

Mustard, Dijon

Mustard, yellow

Nut butter

Nutritional yeast, B_{12}-fortified

Oats, quick

Rice, brown

Seeds, hulled hemp

Soy sauce, low-sodium (or tamari, which is a gluten-free option)

Spirulina

Tempeh, bacon-flavored

Tortillas, whole wheat

Vanilla extract

Vinegar, apple cider

Vinegar, balsamic

Vital wheat gluten

Fresh Produce

Apples, Granny Smith (10)

Avocados (7)

Bananas (2)

Bell peppers, red (2)

Blueberries (24 ounces)

Celery (1 bunch)

Cilantro (1 bunch)

Cucumber (1)

Garlic (1 head)

Ginger (1 root)

Kale (7 cups)

Lemon (1)

Lettuce, romaine (1 head)

Lime (1)

Mushrooms (2 ounces)

Onion, red (1)

Onions, yellow (2)

Oranges, mandarin (8)

Potatoes, yellow (4)

Scallions (1 bunch)

Spinach (22 cups)

Tomatoes (5)

Frozen Produce

Beets, 3 (10-ounce) bags

Blueberries, 2 (16-ounce) bags

Broccoli florets, 5 (16-ounce) bags

Carrots, 1 (16-ounce) bag

Cherries, 1 (16-ounce) bag

Corn, 1 (16-ounce) bag

Edamame, shelled, 5 (10-ounce) bags

Peas, green, 1 (16-ounce) bag

Pineapple, 6 (16-ounce) bags

Spices

Garlic powder

Ginger, ground

Onion powder

Pepper, black

Salt, pink Himalayan

Turmeric

Vegan chick'n bouillon

Vegan poultry seasoning

Other

Plant-based milk, unsweetened,
1 gallon

Tofu, firm, 5 (350-gram) blocks

Yogurt, vegan unsweetened plain
(24 ounces)

Equipment List

Air fryer (or oven)

Blender

Food processor

Mason jars with lids

Nonstick skillets and pots

Parchment paper or silicone sheet

Meal Plan

	MONDAY	TUESDAY	WEDNESDAY	THURSDAY
BREAKFAST	2 slices Ezekiel bread with 2 tablespoons nut butter and 1 tablespoon hemp seeds	2 slices Ezekiel bread with 2 tablespoons nut butter and 1 tablespoon hemp seeds	Tofu Scramble (page 71) with 2 slices of Ezekiel bread	Tofu Scramble with 2 slices of Ezekiel bread
PRE-WORKOUT	Beet Blast Smoothie (page 59)	Beet Blast Smoothie	Beet Blast Smoothie	Banana Protein Pancakes (page 66) with 2 mandarin oranges
POST-WORKOUT	Green Power Smoothie (page 60) *Optional: add 2 tablespoons pea protein powder for 30 grams of additional protein*	Green Power Smoothie *Optional: add 2 tablespoons pea protein powder for 30 grams of additional protein*	Green Power Smoothie *Optional: add 2 tablespoons pea protein powder for 30 grams of additional protein*	Green Power Smoothie *Optional: add 2 tablespoons pea protein powder for 30 grams of additional protein*
LUNCH	Fiesta Black Bean Salad (page 82) (½ portion) with 1 cup shelled edamame	Fiesta Black Bean Salad (½ portion) with 1 cup shelled edamame	Club Wrap with side salad (spinach, tomato, cucumber, green onion, balsamic vinegar)	Chickpea Salad Sandwich (page 92)
SNACK	1 cup vegan yogurt with 1 cup blueberries and ¼ cup raw almonds	1 cup steamed shelled edamame with 1 tablespoon B_{12}-fortified nutritional yeast	1 cup steamed shelled edamame with 1 tablespoon B_{12}-fortified nutritional yeast	1 cup vegan yogurt with 1 cup blueberries and ¼ cup raw almonds
DINNER	Club Wrap (page 93) with side salad (spinach, tomato, cucumber, green onion, balsamic vinegar)	Air-Fried Chicken-Style Seitan (page 127) with baked potato and 2 cups steamed broccoli	Air-Fried Chicken-Style Seitan with baked potato and 2 cups steamed broccoli	Air-Fried Chicken-Style Seitan with baked potato, 1 cup steamed green peas, and 1 cup carrots

	FRIDAY	SATURDAY	SUNDAY
BREAKFAST	Chickpea Omelet (page 68)	Tofu Scramble with 2 slices of Ezekiel bread	Tofu Scramble with 2 slices of Ezekiel bread
PRE-WORKOUT	Banana Protein Pancakes with 2 mandarin oranges	Banana Protein Pancakes with 2 mandarin oranges	Banana Protein Pancakes with 2 mandarin oranges
POST-WORKOUT	Green Power Smoothie *Optional: add 2 tablespoons pea protein powder for 30 grams of additional protein*	Green Power Smoothie *Optional: add 2 tablespoons pea protein powder for 30 grams of additional protein*	Green Power Smoothie *Optional: add 2 tablespoons pea protein powder for 30 grams of additional protein*
LUNCH	Chickpea Salad Sandwich	Chickpea Salad Sandwich	Chickpea Salad Sandwich
SNACK	1 cup steamed shelled edamame with 1 tablespoon B_{12}-fortified nutritional yeast	1 cup vegan yogurt with 1 cup blueberries and ¼ cup raw almonds	1 cup steamed shelled edamame with 1 tablespoon B_{12}-fortified nutritional yeast
DINNER	Maple-Garlic Air-Fried Tofu (page 143) with 1 cup brown rice and 2 cups steamed broccoli	Maple-Garlic Air-Fried Tofu with 1 cup brown rice and 2 cups steamed broccoli	Air-Fried Chicken-Style Seitan with baked potato and 2 cups steamed broccoli

Total Macros and Calories for the Week:

Calories: 16,706

Protein: 990 grams

Carbs: 2,400 grams

Fat: 452 grams

Putting the optional scoop of vegan protein powder in your post-workout smoothie could add up to 30 grams of protein and about 170 calories per day.

Step-by-Step Prep

PREP DAY #1—SUNDAY

Prepare Beet Blast Smoothie (page 59) and Green Power Smoothie (page 60) today and store them in your freezer. Remember, they will take a little bit of time to thaw before drinking, so remove them from the freezer ahead of time. Mason jars are great for storing smoothies.

Vegan unsweetened plain yogurt, blueberries, and almonds are snacks 3 times this week. Portion out each item and store in containers for ready-to-go options.

Steam the edamame for 5 to 7 minutes once the water starts to boil, then store in the refrigerator. You will be having 6 cups this week, and you can eat it warm or cold. Four separate cups are for snacks, and 2 cups are included with each serving of Fiesta Black Bean Salad.

Fiesta Black Bean Salad (page 82) is a 2-serving recipe, so you will divide it in half and store in the refrigerator for lunch on Monday and Tuesday. Remember to include 1 cup of steamed edamame with each of these lunches.

Tofu Scramble (page 71) is a 2-serving recipe, and you are having it 4 times this week. Double the recipe and cook it all at once in a large nonstick skillet. Divide into 4 equal parts and store in the refrigerator in separate containers. You will also include 2 slices of Ezekiel bread with each of the four meals, toasted or as is.

You can prepare Club Wraps (page 93) in advance by separating the ingredients into containers. Don't put the ingredients in the wrap until you are ready to eat or it will get soggy. You can also make the side salad for Monday's and Wednesday's club wraps and store in its own container with the balsamic vinegar kept separate.

Air-Fried Chicken-Style Seitan (page 127) is made in an air fryer, but you can also bake this in the oven at 350°F on parchment paper or a silicone sheet if you don't have an air fryer. You will also be baking 4 potatoes and steaming 6 cups of broccoli, 1 cup of green peas, and 1 cup of carrots. Divide into 4 separate containers and store in the refrigerator.

PREP DAY #2—THURSDAY

Chickpea Omelet (page 68) is for Friday's breakfast. Prepare it and store in a container in the refrigerator.

Prepare a double batch of Banana Protein Pancakes (page 66) so you have 3 pancakes for each of your 4 pre-workout snacks. Remember to grab 2 mandarins per snack, too.

Chickpea Salad Sandwich is a 2-serving recipe. It's on the meal plan 4 times this week, so double the batch. Store it in the refrigerator, and place on the bread when you're ready to eat.

Maple-Garlic Air-Fried Tofu (page 143) is made in an air fryer, but you can also bake it in the oven on parchment paper or a silicone sheet if you don't have an air fryer. You will also be preparing 2 cups of cooked brown rice (1 cup per meal) and 4 cups of steamed broccoli (2 cups per meal). Divide the 2 meals and store in containers in the refrigerator.

Maximizing Recovery

When you finish your workout, it's best to eat within about 30 minutes, the time frame when your muscles are seeking fuel to start the repair process. Although protein is key, so are carbohydrates, because they work best together to stimulate muscles and absorb amino acids. Carbs replenish the glycogen in your muscles and liver, and protein helps your body build and repair muscle cells.

Choose nutrient-dense, easy-to-digest foods that help your body get out of the acidic state. Include alkaline fruits and vegetables such as leafy greens, broccoli, potatoes, bananas, avocados, celery, lime, and quinoa, to name just a few.

It's very important to hydrate before and after activity, and to replenish electrolytes. When you sweat, you lose electrolytes, and you have to replace them. If you don't, you may experience muscle cramping, fatigue, dizziness, or headaches. Try Electrolyte Sports Drink (page 174) for a healthy, natural alternative to store-bought processed products.

SUSTAINING SUPPLEMENTS

Many athletes, nonvegan and vegan alike, use protein powders to top up their protein intake. Protein supplements are a great option for convenience, and there's nothing wrong with incorporating them into your lifestyle. There are several vegan protein powders available, including pea, brown rice, hemp, and soy.

But aim to get all your protein, or at least most of it, directly from whole food, plant-based sources. If you eat enough nutrient-dense calories, you should have no problem reaching your targets.

If you do use protein powders, choose options that are unsweetened or low in sugar (without artificial sweeteners), minimally processed with a short list of simple ingredients, organic, and with a high-quality BCAA profile. It's also great if the powders include greens and probiotics.

Consider supplementing B_{12}, vitamin D, iron, and omega-3 fatty acids, as well. Although you can obtain all of them from nutrient-dense and fortified plant-based food sources, if you don't think you are getting enough, it's okay to supplement.

Adjusting to Fit Your Needs

Everyone is different. Our schedules, preferences, allergies, food sensitivities, and goals are just some factors that determine what and when we eat. You know your body best. If a recipe or meal plan suggestion doesn't work for you, feel free to switch it up. Replace with another recipe on the meal plan, remove the unwanted ingredient, or substitute an ingredient with similar macros.

All the recipes in this cookbook have been developed to provide you with a variety of nourishing, easy, plant-powered meals to help you thrive. I also provide plenty of options for those with special dietary considerations, such as gluten-free, oil-free, refined sugar–free, soy-free, and nut-free dishes, and substitutions are generally easy.

Some quick swaps include changing up the fruits and veggies, switching out the whole wheat flour for gluten-free almond flour, adjusting the amount of spice to suit your taste, or using your favorite plant-based milk in place of the one suggested.

Aside from the ingredients, it is equally important to adjust the portion sizes and daily caloric totals to meet your personalized needs. This can be done by using the formulas provided to determine your nutritional requirements, but always be intuitive and pay close attention to how you feel when consuming certain foods and portion sizes, before and after activity.

To get the absolute most out of this book, I encourage you to customize as much as you like. The important thing is that you enjoy the meals, feel great, and stick to the plan.

You've Got This

Every journey comes with ups and downs. One of the best strategies for conquering your challenges is to stay focused on the goal and appreciate the progress you make along the way. It's important to celebrate the positive milestones you reach. The road to success will have many curves, but it is worth it when you achieve your goals.

The vegan lifestyle offers an abundance of nutrient-rich, delicious foods easily found at your local grocery store. You can reach your athletic goals without compromising your ethics or breaking your budget.

Be kind to yourself as you navigate the new lifestyle changes. It takes time for a new routine to become second nature. Stay consistent and persevere, even if you go off track temporarily or have a slip-up. You are your only true competition. Stay focused on creating the best version of yourself. You've got this!

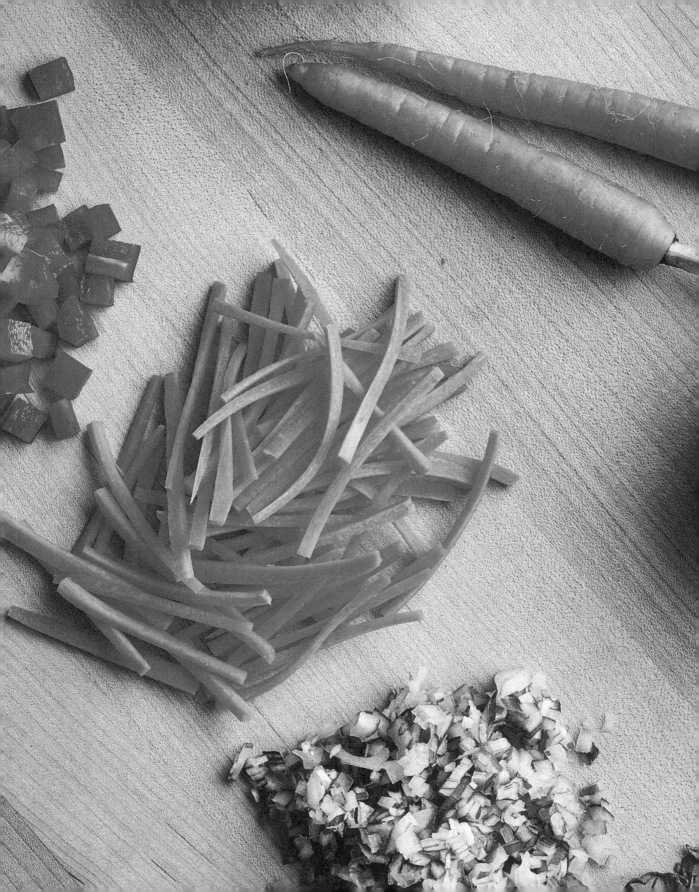

PART 2:

The Recipes

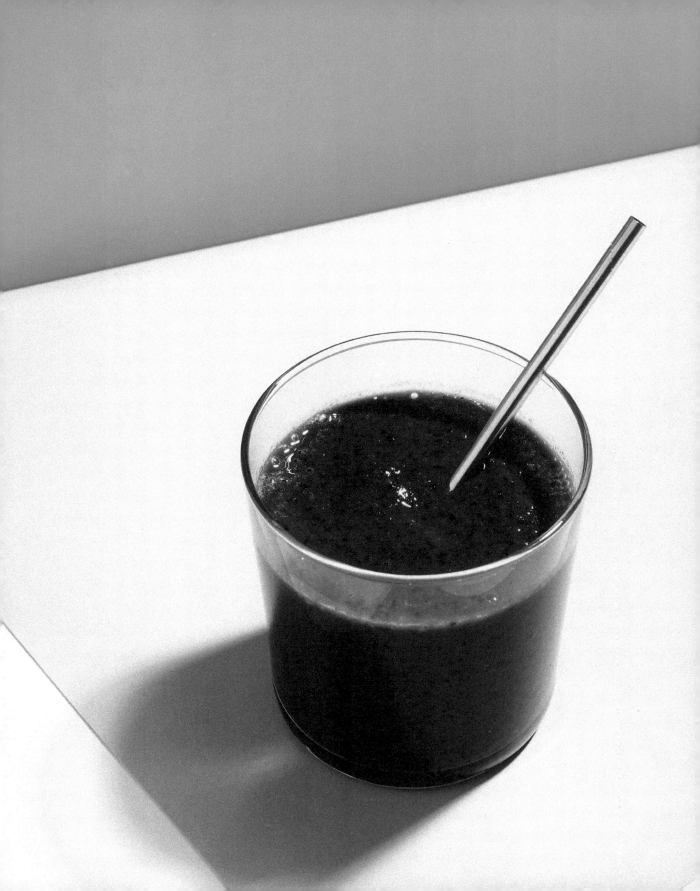

CHAPTER 4

Breakfast and Smoothies

Beet Blast Smoothie, 59

Anti-Inflammatory Juice

Prep time: 15 minutes

SERVES 1

RECOVERY   GLUTEN-FREE   NUT-FREE

This juice packs in the carrots and celery, along with fresh turmeric and ginger, all of which help fight inflammation. Enjoy this nutritious, super-hydrating blend any time to help your body recover from intense training. I love drinking it first thing in the morning.

6 large carrots

3 celery stalks

1 orange, peeled

2-inch fresh ginger root

1-inch fresh
  turmeric root

Juice of 1 lemon

▶ Combine the carrots, celery, orange, ginger, and turmeric in a juicer and turn it on. Squeeze the lemon juice into the finished juice. Enjoy immediately or refrigerate for up to 24 hours.

Per serving: Calories: 285; Total fat: 4g; Carbohydrates: 68g; Fiber: 18g; Protein: 7g; Calcium: 28%; Vitamin D: 0%; Vitamin B$_{12}$: 0%; Iron: 11%; Zinc: 9%

Equipment Tip: You don't need to splurge on expensive juicing machines. There are many budget-friendly juicers available that get the job done.

Beet Blast Smoothie

Prep time: 5 minutes
SERVES 1

PRE-GAME GLUTEN-FREE NUT-FREE

This smoothie provides the benefits of beets with the sweetness of apple, cherries, and blueberries. Beets are a great choice before training because of their high nitrate levels, which help blood flow and blood pressure and can boost athletic performance.

1½ cups unsweetened plant-based milk

1 Granny Smith apple, peeled, cored, and chopped

1 cup chopped frozen beets

1 cup frozen blueberries

½ cup frozen cherries

¼-inch fresh ginger root, peeled

▶ In a blender, combine all the ingredients and blend until smooth. Serve immediately or store in the freezer in a resealable jar.

Per serving: Calories: 324; Total fat: 5g; Carbohydrates: 70g; Fiber: 15g; Protein: 5g; Calcium: 72%; Vitamin D: 38%; Vitamin B_{12}: 0%; Iron: 15%; Zinc: 4%

Prep Tip: Double or triple this recipe. Separate into equal parts and store in Mason jars in the freezer for quick grab-and-go pre-game fuel.

Green Power Smoothie

Prep time: 5 minutes

SERVES 1

RECOVERY GLUTEN-FREE NUT-FREE

Enjoy this smoothie any time. Give it a try as your post-workout fuel because it is packed with kale, spinach, and avocado, all of which help your body get out of an acidic state. This smoothie also includes healthy sources of protein, carbs, and essential fats.

3 cups fresh spinach

1½ cups frozen pineapple

1 cup unsweetened plant-based milk

1 cup fresh kale

1 Granny Smith apple, peeled, cored, and chopped

½ small avocado, pitted and peeled

½ teaspoon spirulina

1 tablespoon hemp seeds

▶ In a blender, combine all the ingredients and blend until smooth. Serve immediately or store in the freezer in a resealable jar.

Per serving: Calories: 431; Total fat: 16g; Carbohydrates: 70g; Fiber: 17g; Protein: 13g; Calcium: 67%; Vitamin D: 25%; Vitamin B$_{12}$: 31%; Iron: 41%; Zinc: 15%

Nutrition Tip: If you want to boost the protein, add 1 scoop of protein powder. Choose a powder that is minimally processed with a short ingredient list, and opt for one that is unsweetened or low in sugar, and free of artificial sweeteners.

Tropical Bliss Smoothie

Prep time: 5 minutes

ENERGY BOOST **GLUTEN-FREE**

SERVES 1

This smoothie brings the beach vibes: the refreshing smell of coconut combined with delicious tropical fruit flavors. Try various combinations by adding different tropical fruits, such as mango, papaya, and passion fruit.

2 cups frozen pineapple

1 banana

1¼ cups unsweetened
  coconut milk

¼ cup frozen
  coconut pieces

½ teaspoon ground
  flaxseed

1 teaspoon hemp seeds

▶ In a blender, combine all the ingredients and blend until smooth. Serve immediately or store in the freezer in a resealable jar.

Per serving: Calories: 396; Total fat: 14g; Carbohydrates: 71g; Fiber: 11g; Protein: 6g; Calcium: 64%; Vitamin D: 31%; Vitamin B$_{12}$: 3%; Iron: 19%; Zinc: 7%

Nutrition Tip: Pineapple contains tons of essential nutrients. Its high vitamin C content helps build a healthy immune system and aids in the absorption of non-heme (plant-based) iron. It's also manganese-rich, which helps the body maintain a healthy metabolism. This amazing fruit is also known to minimize oxidative stress and reduce inflammation, making it a great choice for athletes.

Very Berry Antioxidant Smoothie

Prep time: 5 minutes

SERVES 1

ENERGY BOOST | GLUTEN-FREE | NUT-FREE

Just as its name states, this smoothie is packed with antioxidants from three different berries. Antioxidant-rich foods can protect your cells from the effects of free radicals and help combat premature aging and many diseases. Not only is this smoothie good for you, it tastes amazing, too.

1 banana

1¼ cups unsweetened plant-based milk

½ cup frozen strawberries

½ cup frozen blueberries

½ cup frozen raspberries

3 pitted Medjool dates

1 tablespoon hulled hemp seeds

½ tablespoon ground flaxseed

1 teaspoon ground chia seeds

▶ In a blender, combine all the ingredients and blend until smooth. Serve immediately or store in the freezer in a resealable jar.

Per serving: Calories: 538; Total fat: 11g; Carbohydrates: 111g; Fiber: 21g; Protein: 10g; Calcium: 75%; Vitamin D: 31%; Vitamin B$_{12}$: 8%; Iron: 26%; Zinc: 13%

Nutrition Tip: Frozen fruits are perfect for smoothies. Frozen fruits have many advantages over fresh: they're usually cheaper, they last longer so you're less likely to waste unused food, and they're picked and packed at their prime, which locks in vitamins, minerals, and antioxidants.

Easy Overnight Oats

Prep time: 5 minutes, plus overnight

SERVES 1

GRAB AND GO   **GLUTEN-FREE**

Overnight oats are super versatile. You can customize the toppings and make an unlimited number of flavor combinations. Oats are a naturally gluten-free powerhouse whole grain packed with important vitamins, minerals, antioxidants, and fiber, and they are high in iron, zinc, manganese, phosphorus, magnesium, and vitamin B_1.

½ cup rolled oats (check label for gluten-free)

½ cup unsweetened plant-based milk

1 tablespoon nut butter

½ tablespoon cacao powder

½ teaspoon hulled hemp hearts

½ teaspoon maple syrup

Optional toppings

Dark chocolate chips

Pecans

Strawberries

▶ Combine all the ingredients in a Mason jar or reusable food storage container. Stir together, seal the lid, and place in the refrigerator overnight. When ready to eat, add your favorite toppings.

Per serving: Calories: 347; Total fat: 14g; Carbohydrates: 48g; Fiber: 11g; Protein: 12g; Calcium: 26%; Vitamin D: 13%; Vitamin B_{12}: 1%; Iron: 19%; Zinc: 7%

Prep Tip: These oats store well for up to 5 days in the refrigerator, so if you're planning meals for the week ahead, make a bigger batch and divide into separate containers for a healthy option when you're in a hurry.

Apple-Cinnamon Quinoa

Prep time: 5 minutes
Cook time: 5 minutes

ENERGY BOOST **GLUTEN-FREE**

SERVES 1

Quinoa is a vegan staple. It's a naturally gluten-free, protein-rich seed that comes from the amaranth family. Apple-Cinnamon Quinoa stores well in the refrigerator for 5 to 7 days; make a bigger batch so you can grab it any time. Energize your busy day, fuel your workouts, or support your muscle recovery and growth with this dish.

1½ cups water

1½ cups diced Granny Smith apples

½ cup quinoa, rinsed

1 teaspoon ground flaxseed

½ teaspoon ground cinnamon

Optional toppings

Maple syrup

Nuts and seeds

Nut butter

Fresh fruit

Unsweetened plant-based milk

1. In a medium pot over medium-high heat, combine the water, apples, quinoa, and flaxseed for 5 minutes, or until the water has been fully absorbed.

2. Transfer the quinoa mixture to a bowl and stir in the cinnamon.

3. Serve immediately as is or with your favorite toppings.

Per serving: Calories: 456; Total fat: 7g; Carbohydrates: 90g; Fiber: 12g; Protein: 13g; Calcium: 7%; Vitamin D: 0%; Vitamin B$_{12}$: 0%; Iron: 29%; Zinc: 1%

Nutrition Tip: Quinoa is a high-quality vegan protein source that contains significant amounts of the nine essential amino acids. Quinoa is also a good source of lysine, which is essential for tissue repair and muscle growth.

Strawberry-Kiwi Chia Pudding

Prep time: 5 minutes, plus 4 hours

SERVES 2

PRE-GAME GLUTEN-FREE

Chia pudding is a great fuel for endurance athletes before activity because it provides energy over a longer period by regulating the conversion of carbohydrates. Plus, this pudding is a tasty way to get essential omega-3 fatty acids, protein, iron, calcium, and fiber.

2 cups unsweetened coconut milk, divided

3 Medjool dates, pitted

1 tablespoon vanilla extract

½ cup chia seeds

Toppings

2 kiwis, sliced

4 strawberries, sliced

2 tablespoons unsweetened coconut shreds

2 tablespoons sliced or chopped almonds

1. In a food processor, blend ¾ cup of coconut milk, the dates, and vanilla.

2. Pour the blended mix into a large reusable container or Mason jar. Add the remaining 1¼ cups of coconut milk and the chia seeds. Cover the container and shake gently or stir to mix.

3. Store in the refrigerator overnight or for at least 4 hours, until the chia seeds absorb all the milk. (Optional: stir once or twice as it is setting to avoid clumps.)

4. When ready to eat, top the pudding with the kiwi, strawberries, coconut, and almonds.

5. Store in the refrigerator for up to 5 days.

Per serving: Calories: 783; Total fat: 38g; Carbohydrates: 79g; Fiber: 48g; Protein: 27g; Calcium: 89%; Vitamin D: 60%; Vitamin B_{12}: 100%; Iron: 54%; Zinc: 11%

Substitution Tip: There are so many easy ways to switch up this pudding. Try adding in-season fruits, different plant-based milks, almond slivers, cashews, sunflower seeds, dark chocolate chips, coconut shreds, cinnamon, spirulina, cacao, matcha, or maple syrup. The options are endless.

Banana Protein Pancakes

Prep time: 5 minutes
Cook time: 15 minutes
SERVES 2

STRENGTH BUILDER   NUT-FREE

When I developed this recipe for tasty pancakes, I wanted it to pack a protein punch without using powders. Although powders can be great for convenience, there's no shortage of plant-based foods, such as vital wheat gluten, that can easily boost your protein levels.

1½ cups unsweetened
plant-based milk

1 cup quick oats

1 banana

½ cup vital
wheat gluten

½ cup whole
wheat flour

2 tablespoons
maple syrup

2 teaspoons
vanilla extract

1 teaspoon pink
Himalayan salt

Optional toppings

Sliced bananas

Pecans

Hulled hemp seeds

Maple syrup

1. In a food processor, combine all the ingredients except the optional toppings and mix until smooth.

2. Use a ¼-cup measuring cup to pour ⅙ of the batter into a nonstick skillet over medium heat. Once the edges of the pancake start to brown and bubble, flip and cook the other side. Repeat with the remaining batter.

3. Serve immediately with your favorite toppings (if using) or store the pancakes in the refrigerator in a sealed container for up to 3 days.

Per serving (3 pancakes): Calories: 546; Total fat: 6g; Carbohydrates: 86g; Fiber: 11g; Protein: 36g: Calcium: 42%; Vitamin D: 23%; Vitamin B_{12}: 38%; Iron: 34%; Zinc: 11%

Nutrition Tip: Vital wheat gluten is the flour form of the natural protein found in wheat. It's very high in protein and works beautifully in delicious meat alternatives, such as Air-Fried Chicken-Style Seitan (page 127).

Recipe Tip: You can find vital wheat gluten in the health section of grocery stores or in specialty stores and online.

Blueberry Scones

Prep time: 5 minutes, plus 20 minutes to freeze

Cook time: 25 minutes

SERVES 6

GRAB AND GO

Scones come in all shapes, sizes, and flavors. Blueberry scones have always been my favorite. In addition to their great taste, blueberries are full of antioxidants and packed with nutrients. You can't go wrong.

2 cups whole
   wheat flour
½ cup coconut sugar
2½ teaspoons
   baking powder
½ teaspoon pink
   Himalayan salt

½ cup unsweetened
   applesauce
3 tablespoons aquafaba
   (the liquid from a can
   of chickpeas)

2½ teaspoons
   vanilla extract
⅓ cup chopped
   almonds
1 cup fresh blueberries

1. Preheat the oven to 400°F.

2. In a large bowl, mix the flour, coconut sugar, baking powder, and salt. Add the applesauce, aquafaba, and vanilla and mix the dough together by hand. Gently stir in the almonds and blueberries.

3. Line an 8-inch square baking pan with parchment paper and spread the dough evenly in the pan.

4. Freeze the dough for 20 minutes.

5. Bake for 25 minutes, or until light brown. Once cooled, cut into 6 scones.

6. Store at room temperature in a covered container for up to 5 days.

Per serving: Calories: 265; Total fat: 3g; Carbohydrates: 54g; Fiber: 7g; Protein: 5g; Calcium: 16%; Vitamin D: 0%; Vitamin B_{12}: 0%; Iron: 14%; Zinc: 1%

Recipe Tip: To get a light brown top, combine 1 tablespoon of unsweetened applesauce with 1 tablespoon of unsweetened plant-based milk and brush the top of the scone dough with the mixture before you put it into the oven.

Chickpea Omelet

Prep time: 5 minutes
Cook time: 10 minutes
SERVES 1

STRENGTH BUILDER   **GLUTEN-FREE**   **NUT-FREE**

This omelet is a great way to start your day. Enjoy it as is or with whole-grain toast. Made with high-protein chickpea flour, this omelet delivers on flavor without the cholesterol from eggs.

½ cup chickpea flour
⅛ teaspoon turmeric
⅛ teaspoon pink
  Himalayan salt or
  black salt
⅛ teaspoon freshly
  ground black pepper

⅓ cup water
¼ cup chopped
  mushrooms
¼ cup chopped spinach

¼ cup chopped red
  bell pepper
2 tablespoons diced
  yellow onion
¼ cup vegetable broth

1. In a medium bowl, mix together the chickpea flour, turmeric, salt, and black pepper. Add the water and mix well until smooth.

2. In a medium nonstick pan over medium heat, sauté the mushrooms, spinach, bell pepper, and onion in the vegetable broth for 5 minutes, or until soft.

3. Pour the chickpea mixture into the skillet while there is still some veggie broth remaining. Cook for 5 minutes, or until the edges start to bubble. Fold over the omelet and continue to cook for 3 to 5 minutes, or until lightly browned.

4. Store any leftovers in a reusable container in the refrigerator for up to 3 days.

Per serving: Calories: 206; Total fat: 3g; Carbohydrates: 32g; Fiber: 7g; Protein: 12g; Calcium: 4%; Vitamin D: 3%; Vitamin B$_{12}$: <1%; Iron: 16%; Zinc: 10%

Recipe Tip: Optional toppings include avocado slices, salsa, black beans, freshly diced tomatoes, or vegan cheese.

Cinnamon French Toast

Prep time: 5 minutes

Cook time: 10 minutes

SERVES 2

A childhood favorite, veganized! No need for eggs to enjoy a great French toast. This flavorful recipe is perfect for breakfast or whenever your sweet tooth needs a fix. The mixture stores well in the refrigerator for up to 3 days.

1 cup unsweetened plant-based milk

¾ cup firm tofu

½ teaspoon vanilla extract

½ teaspoon ground cinnamon

¼ teaspoon ground flaxseed

4 slices thick whole wheat bread

1. In a blender, blend the milk, tofu, vanilla, cinnamon, and flaxseed until smooth.
2. Pour the mixture into a wide bowl. Dip the bread slices into the mixture until evenly coated on both sides.
3. In a medium nonstick pan over medium heat, cook the bread slices, flipping when the bottom is light brown. Flip again, if needed.

Per serving: Calories: 642; Total fat: 20g; Carbohydrates: 92g; Fiber: 14g; Protein: 31g; Calcium: 230%; Vitamin D: 25%; Vitamin B_{12}: 0%; Iron: 40%; Zinc: 38%

Recipe Tip: Add your favorite toppings, such as maple syrup, fresh fruit, nut butter, nuts, or seeds.

Mango Coconut Rice

Prep time: 5 minutes

Cook time: 30 minutes

SERVES 2

GRAB AND GO GLUTEN-FREE

Mango coconut rice is a traditional Thai dessert, but this recipe makes a great breakfast or snack, too. This rice is topped with fresh mango, but you can use different tropical fruits, nuts, and seeds to switch it up from time to time.

2 cups canned
  coconut milk
1 cup brown rice

1 cup water
¼ cup maple syrup
1 cup cubed mango

Cashews (optional)

1. In a medium nonstick pan over medium-high heat, combine the coconut milk, rice, water, and maple syrup. Bring to a boil, cover, and reduce the heat to low. Cook for 30 minutes, or until the rice is soft and thickened. Remove from the heat and let it cool.

2. Top with the mango and cashews (if using).

Per serving: Calories: 901; Total fat: 46g; Carbohydrates: 120g; Fiber: 6g; Protein: 12g; Calcium: 4%; Vitamin D: 0%; Vitamin B$_{12}$: 0%; Iron: 17%; Zinc: 11%

Prep Tip: Feel free to make a larger batch and store it in the refrigerator for up to 5 days so it's ready when you are.

Tofu Scramble

Prep time: 5 minutes
Cook time: 15 minutes
SERVES 2

STRENGTH BUILDER **GLUTEN-FREE** **NUT-FREE**

This tasty vegan alternative to scrambled eggs is protein-rich and cholesterol-free. Enjoy it alone or with toast, or satisfy a big appetite by eating it with a stack of Banana Protein Pancakes (page 66).

½ yellow onion, diced
½ red bell pepper, diced
1 (350-gram) block
   firm tofu

½ cup unsweetened
   plant-based milk
¼ teaspoon turmeric

¼ teaspoon freshly
   ground black pepper

1. In a nonstick pan over medium heat, sauté the onion and bell pepper in a little bit of water for 3 to 5 minutes, or until soft. Break the tofu into small pieces and add it to the pan along with the milk, turmeric, and black pepper. Stir together and continue to cook for another 8 to 10 minutes.

2. Serve immediately or store in a reusable container in the refrigerator for up to 3 days.

Per serving: Calories: 214; Total fat: 10g; Carbohydrates: 12g; Fiber: 4g; Protein: 22g; Calcium: 26%; Vitamin D: 6%; Vitamin B_{12}: 0%; Iron: 22%; Zinc: 1%

Recipe Tip: You can add more vegetables, such as spinach, mushrooms, or kale, to your tofu scramble. Wrap in a whole wheat tortilla to enjoy it on the go.

Country Breakfast Skillet

Prep time: 10 minutes
Cook time: 45 minutes

SERVES 2

STRENGTH BUILDER **GLUTEN-FREE** **NUT-FREE**

This recipe is a hearty meal for those who wake up with a big appetite. Packed with potatoes, vegetables, tempeh, and tofu, this breakfast dish is low in fat and big on flavor.

For the potatoes

2 tablespoons
    vegetable broth
¼ teaspoon
    garlic powder
¼ teaspoon freshly
    ground black pepper
⅛ teaspoon pink
    Himalayan salt

3 yellow
    potatoes, chopped

For the skillet

1 tablespoon paprika
¼ teaspoon freshly
    ground black pepper
⅛ teaspoon pink
    Himalayan salt

⅛ teaspoon turmeric
3 cups baby spinach
½ (350-gram) block firm
    tofu, cubed
6 slices bacon-flavored
    tempeh, chopped
¼ cup vegetable broth
1 yellow onion, chopped
1 red bell pepper, diced
3 garlic cloves, minced

To make the potatoes

1. Preheat the oven to 400°F. Line a baking sheet with parchment paper or a silicone liner.

2. In a large bowl, mix the broth, garlic powder, pepper, and salt. Add the potatoes and mix well.

3. Spread the potatoes on the prepared baking sheet and bake for 30 minutes, or until soft and browned on the edges.

To make the skillet

4. In a small bowl, mix the paprika, black pepper, salt, and turmeric.

5. In a large nonstick skillet over medium heat, combine the spinach, tofu, tempeh, broth, onion, bell pepper, and garlic. Stir in the seasoning mix. Cover the skillet and cook for 5 minutes. Add the cooked potatoes and cook, stirring frequently, for another 5 minutes.

6. Serve immediately or store in the refrigerator in a sealed container for up to 3 days.

Per serving: Calories: 433; Total fat: 8g; Carbohydrates: 68g; Fiber: 14g; Protein: 27g; Calcium: 24%; Vitamin D: 0%; Vitamin B$_{12}$: 0%; Iron: 46%; Zinc: 6%

Nutrition Tip: Tempeh is fermented, so it promotes the growth of good gut bacteria, known as probiotics, that help digestion, immune function, and heart health.

Substitution Tip: Try swapping out the yellow potatoes for sweet potatoes to add extra fiber and antioxidants.

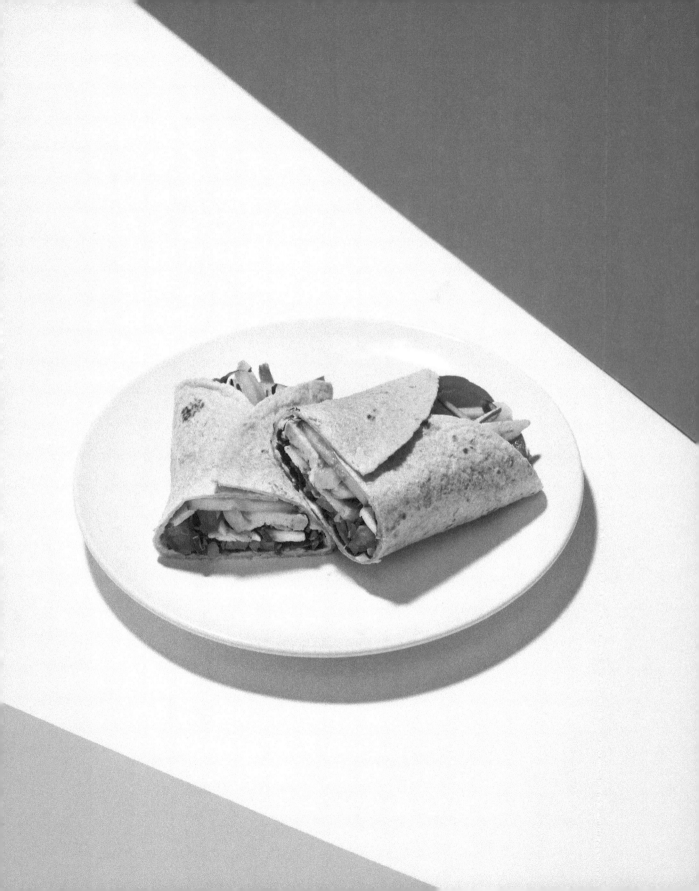

Midday Meals

Veggie Rainbow Wrap, 94

Air-Fried Spring Rolls

Prep time: 20 minutes

Cook time: 12 minutes, then 6 minutes per batch to air fry

MAKES 15 SPRING ROLLS

If you're looking for something to bring to a potluck or serve as an appetizer, Air-Fried Spring Rolls are the way to go. They make an incredible snack, too. Whenever I make these spring rolls, they disappear in a flash.

3 garlic cloves, minced

1 teaspoon minced peeled fresh ginger

¼ cup vegetable broth

2 cups shredded cabbage

1½ cups diced shiitake mushrooms

1 cup shredded carrots

½ cup diced firm tofu

1 scallion, diced

1 tablespoon low-sodium soy sauce (or tamari, which is a gluten-free option)

14 to 16 vegan spring roll pastry sheets

Sweet Ginger Sauce (page 176), for dipping (optional)

1. In a large nonstick pan over medium heat, sauté the garlic and ginger in the broth for 2 minutes, or until softened. Add the cabbage, mushrooms, carrots, tofu, scallion, and soy sauce. Stir, cover the pan, and continue to sauté for 10 minutes, stirring frequently.

2. Form the spring rolls. Place 1 generous tablespoon of the mixture in the middle of a pastry sheet. Roll and fold in the ends. Dab your finger in water and glue the ends closed. Repeat with the remaining mixture and pastry sheets.

3. Place the spring rolls in the air fryer and cook for 6 minutes, or until lightly browned on the edges. (Air fryer machines vary, so keep your eye on it to avoid burning.)

4. Enjoy immediately with sweet ginger sauce (if using) or store in a reusable container in the refrigerator for up to 5 days.

Per serving (1 roll): Calories: 59; Total fat: <1g; Carbohydrates: 13g; Fiber: 1g; Protein: 2g; Calcium: 7%; Vitamin D: 0%; Vitamin B$_{12}$: 0%; Iron: 2%; Zinc: 3%

Recipe Tip: To reheat spring rolls, put them on a baking sheet lined with parchment paper or a silicone liner in a preheated oven at 350°F for 5 to 7 minutes.

Substitution Tip: This recipe uses an air fryer, but you can also bake the spring rolls on a baking sheet lined with parchment paper or a silicone liner in a preheated oven at 350°F for 20 to 30 minutes, or until the edges are browned. The results won't be exactly the same, but they will still turn out well.

Greek Stuffed Avocado

Prep time: 5 minutes, plus 1 hour to marinate

SERVES 1

Avocados and black olives are healthy sources of the essential fats our bodies require. Most of the fat in the avocado fruit is oleic acid, which has been associated with reducing inflammation. Avocado also has more potassium than bananas and is high in vitamins C, K, E, and folate. Avocados are all-stars in the vegan athlete's kitchen.

½ (350-gram) block firm tofu, cubed

¼ cup freshly squeezed lemon juice

2 tablespoons unsweetened plant-based milk

1 tablespoon apple cider vinegar

½ tablespoon dried oregano

1 teaspoon B_{12}-fortified nutritional yeast

¼ teaspoon pink Himalayan salt

Pinch freshly ground black pepper

1 large avocado

4 cherry tomatoes, diced

½ small red onion, diced

½ small cucumber, diced

1 tablespoon sliced black olives

1. In a reusable container with a lid, combine the tofu, lemon juice, milk, vinegar, oregano, nutritional yeast, salt, and pepper. Cover and gently shake to mix. Marinate in the refrigerator for at least 1 hour.

2. Cut the avocado in half, remove the pit, and stuff both halves with the tomatoes, onion, cucumber, olives, and tofu feta. Serve immediately.

Per serving: Calories: 603; Total fat: 41g; Carbohydrates: 43g; Fiber: 21g; Protein: 29g; Calcium: 29%; Vitamin D: 3%; Vitamin B_{12}: 17%; Iron: 36%; Zinc: 7%

Recipe Tip: The longer you marinate the tofu feta, the more flavorful it will become. Try preparing this the night before you want to eat it so the flavors can meld overnight.

Alkaline Protein Power Salad

Prep time: 5 minutes

SERVES 2

ENERGY BOOST   **GLUTEN-FREE**   **NUT-FREE**

For many years this has been one of my go-to meals before or after Tae Kwon Do and hockey. This salad is satisfying and nutritious and provides sustainable energy without weighing me down. I highly recommend adding this meal on your active days. It is easily digestible and contains health-promoting protein, carbs, and essential fats.

4 cups chopped kale

2 tablespoons freshly
    squeezed lemon juice

⅛ teaspoon pink
    Himalayan salt

1 cup cooked wild rice

1 cup cooked quinoa

1 small tomato, chopped

1 small avocado, pitted,
    peeled, and chopped

1. In a large bowl, massage the kale with the lemon juice and salt for a few minutes, or until the kale softens.

2. Add the rice, quinoa, tomato, and avocado to the bowl and mix well.

3. Enjoy immediately or store in the refrigerator for up to 3 days.

Per serving: Calories: 722; Total fat: 20g; Carbohydrates: 123g; Fiber: 28g; Protein: 27g; Calcium: 40%; Vitamin D: 0%; Vitamin B_{12}: 0%; Iron: 53%; Zinc: 28%

Nutrition Tip: You should eat plenty of foods that help your body stay in an alkaline state, as opposed to those that put your body into an acidic state. This includes plant-based foods, like the ingredients in this recipe, that are closest to their natural state, are not highly processed, and don't cause inflammation in the body.

Mediterranean Couscous Salad

Prep time: 10 minutes

Cook time: 10 minutes

SERVES 1

Couscous is made by moistening coarsely ground durum wheat and tossing it with fine wheat flour until it forms tiny balls. It's rich in selenium, which is a powerful antioxidant that helps your body decrease inflammation and repair damaged cells. This salad is an adaptation of the one I ate as a child. Couscous has a pleasant fluffy texture, and it absorbs all the other flavors in the dish.

1½ cups water

1 cup couscous

½ cup cooked chickpeas (drained and rinsed, if canned)

½ small red bell pepper, chopped

1 small red onion, diced

½ cucumber, chopped

1 small tomato, chopped

1 scallion, chopped

1 tablespoon balsamic vinegar

⅛ teaspoon pink Himalayan salt

⅛ teaspoon freshly ground black pepper

1. In a nonstick pot over medium-high heat, bring the water to a boil. Add the couscous. Turn off the heat, stir the couscous, and cover. Let it sit for 5 minutes, until the couscous has fully absorbed the water and is soft.

2. Transfer the couscous to a bowl. Add the chickpeas, bell pepper, onion, cucumber, tomato, scallion, vinegar, salt, and black pepper. Mix well. Serve immediately or store in a reusable container in the refrigerator for up to 7 days.

Per serving: Calories: 822; Total fat: 3g; Carbohydrates: 170g; Fiber: 17g; Protein: 29g; Calcium: 14%; Vitamin D: 0%; Vitamin B$_{12}$: 0%; Iron: 28%; Zinc: 22%

Recipe Tip: Drizzle Italian Hemp Dressing (page 179) on top, mix, and enjoy.

Super Spinach Chickpea Salad

Prep time: 10 minutes

STRENGTH BUILDER **GLUTEN-FREE** **NUT-FREE**

SERVES 1

Spinach is a leafy green that is high in vitamin C, which helps your body boost its absorption of the iron in the chickpeas. This is key for athletes, who require more iron than sedentary folks. We lose significant amounts of this mineral when we're active, and we have to replenish it. This recipe is a super way to do so.

3 cups baby spinach, roughly chopped

2 cups cooked chickpeas (drained and rinsed, if canned)

1 cup chopped mushrooms

1 tomato, chopped

1 avocado, peeled, pitted, and chopped

⅛ teaspoon pink Himalayan salt

⅛ teaspoon freshly ground black pepper

Juice of 1 large lemon

1 tablespoon sunflower seeds, for topping (optional)

1 teaspoon hulled hemp seeds, for topping (optional)

1. In a large bowl, combine the spinach, chickpeas, mushrooms, tomato, and avocado. Add the salt, pepper, and lemon juice. Mix thoroughly so all the flavors combine and the avocado is mixed in well.

2. Top with the seeds (if using). Enjoy immediately or store in a reusable container in the refrigerator for up to 5 days.

Per serving: Calories: 943; Total fat: 33g; Carbohydrates: 140g; Fiber: 38g; Protein: 34g; Calcium: 34%; Vitamin D: 13%; Vitamin B$_{12}$: 1%; Iron: 70%; Zinc: 45%

Prep Tip: This recipe makes an excellent source of fuel for any time of day, before or after training. Make a larger batch and add it to your meal plan for the week.

Recipe Tip: Try adding ½ cup of cooked quinoa, which goes great with this salad.

Fiesta Black Bean Salad

Prep time: 5 minutes

ENERGY BOOST **GLUTEN-FREE** **NUT-FREE**

SERVES 2

The vegan lifestyle can be budget-friendly when you stick to the staples like beans, lentils, and potatoes. This recipe, like many in this cookbook, proves you don't need to spend a lot of money or search for hard-to-find ingredients to enjoy tasty and nutritious meals.

2 cups cooked black beans (drained and rinsed, if canned)

1 avocado, pitted, peeled, and chopped

½ cup corn (drained and rinsed, if canned)

1 small tomato, chopped

2 scallions, chopped

2 tablespoons diced jalapeños

⅛ cup chopped fresh cilantro

1 tablespoon freshly squeezed lime juice

Pink Himalayan salt (optional)

▶ In a large bowl, combine the beans, avocado, corn, tomato, scallions, jalapeños, and cilantro and mix well with a wooden spoon. Sprinkle with the lime juice and a pinch of salt (if using) and enjoy.

Per serving: Calories: 855; Total fat: 30g; Carbohydrates: 123g; Fiber: 46g; Protein: 38g; Calcium: 18%; Vitamin D: 0%; Vitamin B_{12}: 0%; Iron: 55%; Zinc: 38%

Prep Tip: This recipe is perfect for meal prep. Make a larger batch, divide it into equal parts, and store it in individual reusable containers in the refrigerator for up to 5 days.

Pesto Pasta Salad

Prep time: 5 minutes

SERVES 4

PRE-GAME   GLUTEN-FREE   NUT-FREE

Pesto is an Italian sauce traditionally made with basil, cheese, and oil. In this plant-strong version, there's no cheese or oil but absolutely no compromise on flavor. This pesto pasta salad tastes so fresh. It's a great way to get your fix of healthy leafy greens.

2½ cups fresh basil

2 cups fresh spinach

1 cup chopped
   fresh kale

4 garlic cloves

4 tablespoons freshly
   squeezed lemon juice

¼ teaspoon salt

⅛ teaspoon freshly
   ground black pepper

1 cup sunflower seeds

8 ounces cooked
   chickpea-based pasta
   or whole wheat pasta

1½ cups chopped
   fresh tomatoes

1. In a food processor, combine the basil, spinach, kale, garlic, lemon juice, salt, and pepper, and pulse until lightly blended. Add the sunflower seeds and mix until blended well.

2. In a large bowl, combine the pesto sauce with the cooked pasta and mix well. Top with the tomatoes and enjoy. This stores well in a reusable container in the refrigerator for up to 5 days.

Per serving: Calories: 418; Total fat: 20g; Carbohydrates: 48g; Fiber: 14g; Protein: 23g; Calcium: 15%; Vitamin D: 0%; Vitamin B_{12}: 0%; Iron: 47%; Zinc: 15%

Recipe Tip: Enjoy this dish as is, warm or cold, or try optional toppings, such as avocado, green peas, black olives, or Parmesan Cheese (page 183).

Air-Fried Cauliflower with Bold Barbecue Sauce

Prep time: 10 minutes
Cook time: 15 minutes

SERVES 4

GRAB AND GO | GLUTEN-FREE | NUT-FREE

This recipe is one of my favorite ways to enjoy cauliflower. These bites aren't trying to be chicken wings; they are amazing in their own right. The coating and sauce make them a crowd-pleaser and a go-to option for parties, potlucks, or even a healthy snack.

For the cauliflower

¾ cup plus
  2 tablespoons
  unsweetened
  plant-based milk
¾ cup gluten-free flour
1 teaspoon smoked
  paprika
⅛ teaspoon freshly
  ground black pepper
⅛ teaspoon pink
  Himalayan salt

1 whole cauliflower
  head, chopped into
  2-inch pieces

For the Bold Barbecue Sauce

1 cup ketchup
1 tablespoon apple
  cider vinegar
1 tablespoon
  maple syrup

1 tablespoon molasses
1 tablespoon vegan
  Worcestershire
  sauce (check label
  for gluten-free)
¼ teaspoon
  onion powder
¼ teaspoon
  garlic powder
¼ teaspoon freshly
  ground black pepper

To make the cauliflower

1. In a large bowl, combine the milk, flour, paprika, pepper, and salt. Add the cauliflower and stir to evenly coat the pieces with the mixture.

2. In the air fryer, cook the coated cauliflower pieces for 8 to 12 minutes, or until light golden brown. (Air fryer machines vary, so keep your eye on it to avoid burning.)

To make the sauce

3. In a small bowl, combine all the ingredients and stir to mix well.

4. In a large bowl, combine the cooked cauliflower pieces and sauce, and toss or stir to coat the cauliflower.

Per serving: Calories: 309; Total fat: 2g; Carbohydrates: 70g; Fiber: 8g; Protein: 7g; Calcium: 22%; Vitamin D: 7%; Vitamin B$_{12}$: 0%; Iron: 15%; Zinc: 6%

Recipe Tip: This recipe uses an air fryer, but if you don't have one, you can bake the cauliflower on a baking sheet lined with parchment paper or a silicone liner in a preheated oven at 350°F for 20 to 30 minutes. The results won't be exactly the same as the air-fried version, but the dish will still turn out well.

Substitution Tip: You can toss the cauliflower wings in lots of different sauces. Try a buffalo sauce or Ranch Dressing (page 180).

Buddha Power Bowl

Prep time: 10 minutes
Cook time: 15 minutes
SERVES 1

ENERGY BOOST GLUTEN-FREE OPTION

NUT-FREE

Buddha bowls are simply big bowls packed with a delicious variety of healthy ingredients. This colorful bowl with its ginger-tahini sauce provides a wide range of nutrients in a satisfying meal that will fill you up without making you feel weighed down.

For the vegetables

1 small sweet
   potato, cubed
Freshly ground
   black pepper
Pink Himalayan salt
2 packed cups stemmed
   and chopped kale
½ cup edamame
1 small bunch broccolini
1 avocado, pitted,
   peeled, and sliced
½ cup cooked quinoa

For the ginger-tahini sauce

1-inch fresh ginger
   root, minced
1 garlic clove, minced
2 tablespoons tahini
2 tablespoons water
1 tablespoon freshly
   squeezed lemon juice
½ tablespoon red
   wine vinegar

½ teaspoon
   low-sodium soy sauce
   (or tamari, which is a
   gluten-free option)

Optional toppings

½ cup cooked
   chickpeas (drained
   and rinsed, if canned)
½ cup shredded
   purple cabbage
1 tablespoon shelled
   pumpkin seeds

To make the vegetables

1. Preheat the oven to 400°F. Line a baking sheet with parchment paper or a silicone liner.

2. Spread out the sweet potato on the prepared baking sheet and sprinkle evenly with the pepper and salt. Cook for 15 minutes, or until lightly browned.

3. Steam the kale, edamame, and broccolini for 5 to 7 minutes, or until softened.

To make the ginger-tahini sauce

4. In a medium bowl, combine all the ingredients and mix well.

5. To finish the dish, in a large bowl, arrange the vegetables and the avocado over the quinoa and drizzle with the sauce. Sprinkle with the toppings (if using).

Per serving: Calories: 946; Total fat: 49g; Carbohydrates: 107g; Fiber: 30g; Protein: 32g; Calcium: 51%; Vitamin D: 0%; Vitamin B$_{12}$: 0%; Iron: 59%; Zinc: 24%

Prep Tip: This recipe works well for meal prep, so double or triple it and divide into separate containers. Store in the refrigerator for up to 5 days. Keep the sauce on the side and drizzle it on top when you're ready to eat.

Veggie Sushi Bowl

Prep time: 15 minutes

SERVES 1

ENERGY BOOST   **GLUTEN-FREE**   **NUT-FREE**

This easy and quick recipe deconstructs the traditional veggie sushi roll and puts it in a bowl. You get all the flavorful nutrition without having to make the rolls.

1 cup cooked brown rice

1 small avocado, pitted, peeled, and cut into strips

½ cup shelled edamame

½ cup thinly sliced carrots

½ cucumber, cut into thin strips

1 scallion, chopped

½ nori sheet, cut into thin strips

Low-sodium soy sauce (or tamari, which is gluten-free), for topping (optional)

Pickled ginger, for topping (optional)

Black sesame seeds, for topping (optional)

Wasabi, for a spicy topping (optional)

▶ Put the rice in a serving bowl and layer on the avocado, edamame, carrots, cucumber, scallion, and nori. Add your toppings of choice (if using). Enjoy immediately or store in a reusable container in the refrigerator for up to 5 days. (If storing the rice and vegetables in the refrigerator, don't add the avocado or soy sauce until you're ready to eat.)

Per serving: Calories: 664; Total fat: 32g; Carbohydrates: 81g; Fiber: 21g; Protein: 21g; Calcium: 16%; Vitamin D: 0%; Vitamin B$_{12}$: 0%; Iron: 22%; Zinc: 11%

Nutrition Tip: Nori is an edible seaweed that becomes dark green when dried. It provides a rich supply of iron, iodine, folate, and vitamins K and A, and is low in calories and fat.

Caesar Salad

Prep time: 10 minutes, plus at least
   1 hour to soak the cashews

Cook time: 20 minutes

SERVES 4

Caesar salads are notoriously unhealthy. This veganized version smashes that reputation by using whole food, plant-based ingredients to make a creamy dressing and roasted garlic chickpea croutons that don't sacrifice flavor.

For the croutons

1 (19-ounce) can
   chickpeas, drained
   and rinsed

1 teaspoon
   garlic powder

½ teaspoon
   dried oregano

¼ teaspoon B_{12}-fortified
   nutritional yeast

⅛ teaspoon pink
   Himalayan salt

⅛ teaspoon freshly
   ground black pepper

For the dressing

½ cup raw cashews,
   soaked in hot water for
   at least 1 hour

¼ cup plus
   2 tablespoons
   unsweetened
   plant-based milk

2 garlic cloves

3 tablespoons freshly
   squeezed lemon juice

½ tablespoon
   Dijon mustard

2 teaspoons capers

½ teaspoon vegan
   Worcestershire
   sauce (check label
   for gluten-free)

⅛ teaspoon pink
   Himalayan salt

¼ teaspoon freshly
   ground black pepper

For the salad

1 medium head romaine
   lettuce, chopped

1 small bunch
   kale, chopped

Parmesan Cheese
   (page 183) (optional)

To make the croutons

1. Preheat the oven to 450°F. Line a baking sheet with parchment paper or a silicone liner.

2. Rinse the chickpeas, but do not dry them.

(continued)

Caesar Salad (continued)

3. In a large bowl, combine the garlic powder, oregano, nutritional yeast, salt, and pepper and mix well. Add the chickpeas and mix thoroughly.

4. Spread out the chickpeas evenly on the prepared baking sheet and cook for 20 minutes, or until lightly browned. Roll the chickpeas around at the 10-minute mark. Ovens differ, so keep an eye on the chickpeas to ensure they don't burn.

To make the dressing

5. In a food processor, combine all the ingredients and blend until creamy and completely smooth.

To assemble the salad

6. In a large bowl, combine the romaine lettuce and kale. Top with the roasted garlic chickpea croutons, dressing, and Parmesan cheese (if using). Serve immediately or store the ingredients separately in sealed containers in the refrigerator for up to 3 days.

Per serving: Calories: 277; Total fat: 10g; Carbohydrates: 40g; Fiber: 8g; Protein: 11g; Calcium: 15%; Vitamin D: 2%; Vitamin B$_{12}$: 1%; Iron: 21%; Zinc: 17%

Recipe Tip: Eat this nutritious salad on its own or enjoy it as a side with Spaghetti & Meat-Free Meatballs (page 153).

Tabbouleh

Prep time: 10 minutes
Cook time: 10 minutes
SERVES 2

ENERGY BOOST   **GLUTEN-FREE OPTION**
NUT-FREE

This is the traditional Lebanese recipe I grew up with. It's loaded with fresh ingredients and just a little bulgur wheat. Parsley is rich in vitamins A, C, and K. It's also high in nitrates, which are especially beneficial for athletes because they help dilate blood vessels, which improves blood flow.

⅓ cup water

2 tablespoons
 bulgur wheat

3 cups chopped
 fresh parsley

1 small tomato,
 finely chopped

½ small cucumber,
 finely chopped,
 seeds removed

1 scallion,
 finely chopped

¼ cup chopped fresh
 mint leaves

¼ cup freshly squeezed
 lemon juice

¼ teaspoon pink
 Himalayan salt

1. In a small nonstick pot over high heat, bring the water to a boil, then add the bulgur wheat. Stir continuously for 1 minute. Turn off the heat and continue stirring until the bulgur wheat is tender and has aborbed all the water. Remove from the heat.

2. In a big bowl, combine the bulgur with the remaining ingredients. This stores well in the refrigerator for up to 5 days.

Per serving: Calories: 94; Total fat: 1g; Carbohydrates: 20g; Fiber: 6g; Protein: 5g; Calcium: 16%; Vitamin D: 0%; Vitamin B$_{12}$: 0%; Iron: 38%; Zinc: 10%

Substitution Tip: To make this tabbouleh gluten-free, swap out the bulgur for an equal amount of quinoa.

Chickpea Salad Sandwich

Prep time: 5 minutes
SERVES 2

STRENGTH BUILDER **GLUTEN-FREE OPTION**

Many of us grew up eating egg salad sandwiches, and this Chickpea Salad Sandwich is the perfect replacement. I add tofu into the mix because it creates a similar texture to egg salad that really absorbs the flavors, and it boosts the protein level when combined with the chickpeas.

2 cups cooked
  chickpeas (drained
  and rinsed, if canned)
½ (350-gram) block firm
  tofu, chopped
1 celery stalk, chopped
1 scallion, chopped

3 heaping tablespoons
  Mighty Mayo
  (page 182)
1 tablespoon
  yellow mustard
⅛ teaspoon freshly
  ground black pepper

Pink Himalayan
  salt (optional)
4 slices whole
  wheat bread (or
  gluten-free bread)

1. In a large bowl, mash the chickpeas.
2. Add the tofu, celery, scallion, mayo, mustard, pepper, and salt (if using) and mix well.
3. Spread the salad equally on 2 slices of bread and top with the remaining slices to make 2 sandwiches. This also stores well in a reusable container in the refrigerator for up to 5 days.

Per serving: Calories: 619; Total fat: 15g; Carbohydrates: 94g; Fiber: 19g; Protein: 33g; Calcium: 19%; Vitamin D: 2%; Vitamin B$_{12}$: 0%; Iron: 41%; Zinc: 30%

Nutrition Tip: Use Ezekiel or sprouted grain bread to increase the protein and nutritional benefits. For a lighter option, swap out the bread and make it a lettuce wrap.

Club Wrap

Prep time: 10 minutes

Cook time: 5 minutes

SERVES 1

GRAB AND GO **GLUTEN-FREE**

This wrap is the veganized take on the club sandwich, topped with Mighty Mayo. You can serve it warm or cold—it a great lunch either way.

¼ (350-gram) block firm tofu, sliced

3 slices bacon-flavored tempeh

1 large gluten-free tortilla wrap

1 tablespoon Mighty Mayo (page 182)

1 small avocado, pitted, peeled, and chopped

1 romaine lettuce leaf, chopped

1 small tomato, sliced

¼ small red onion, sliced

⅛ teaspoon freshly ground black pepper

1. Preheat a nonstick pan over medium heat. Place the tofu slices and tempeh in the pan and cook for 3 to 5 minutes, until both sides are lightly browned.

2. Place the tortilla on a plate and spread with the mayo. Layer on the avocado, lettuce, tomato, and onion. Top with the tofu and tempeh and sprinkle with the pepper. Wrap the tortilla and enjoy.

Per serving: Calories: 578; Total fat: 30g; Carbohydrates: 60g; Fiber: 15g; Protein: 23g; Calcium: 22%; Vitamin D: 1%; Vitamin B_{12}: 0%; Iron: 31%; Zinc: 8%

Substitution Tip: For a lighter option, try a lettuce wrap.

Veggie Rainbow Wrap

Prep time: 10 minutes
SERVES 1

GRAB AND GO | GLUTEN-FREE OPTION

NUT-FREE

This Veggie Rainbow Wrap is a bright mix of healthy vegetables and creamy Turmeric Hummus. Eating a variety of colorful foods is a surefire way to ensure you are consuming a wide range of essential nutrients. This wrap is loaded with antioxidants, vitamins, and minerals. It's perfect for athletes on the go.

6 tablespoons Turmeric Hummus (page 184)

1 gluten-free wrap, large flatbread, or whole wheat tortilla

1 cup baby spinach

1 small tomato, diced

1 small avocado, pitted, peeled, and sliced

½ small cucumber, sliced

¼ small yellow bell pepper, chopped

¼ cup shredded carrots

¼ cup sliced mushrooms

¼ cup purple cabbage

Freshly ground black pepper

▶ Spread the hummus on the wrap and layer on the spinach, tomato, avocado, cucumber, bell pepper, carrots, mushrooms, and cabbage and season with pepper. Roll up the wrap and eat immediately or store in a sealed container in the refrigerator for up to 2 days.

Per serving: Calories: 609; Total fat: 34g; Carbohydrates: 65g; Fiber: 17g; Protein: 14g; Calcium: 24%; Vitamin D: 3%; Vitamin B_{12}: <1%; Iron: 35%; Zinc: 8%

Prep Tip: Make more than one wrap at a time to prep your lunch for the next day.

TVP Burritos

Prep time: 10 minutes
Cook time: 10 minutes
SERVES 4

STRENGTH BUILDER   **GLUTEN-FREE**   **NUT-FREE**

Packed with plant-based protein, healthy carbs, and fresh Tex-Mex flavors, this is one of my favorite easy meals. These TVP Burritos are a tasty way to fuel your hardworking muscles. If you don't have tortillas on hand, enjoy the ingredients as a burrito bowl.

For the seasoning

1 tablespoon
   chili powder
1 teaspoon paprika
1 teaspoon
   ground cumin
½ teaspoon
   garlic powder
½ teaspoon
   onion powder
¼ teaspoon freshly
   ground black pepper
¼ teaspoon red
   pepper flakes

⅛ teaspoon
   dried oregano
⅛ teaspoon salt

For the burritos

1 cup vegetable broth
¼ cup water
1 cup dried
   TVP (textured
   vegetable protein)
4 large gluten-free
   tortillas
2 cups cooked
   brown rice

2 cups cooked black
   beans (drained and
   rinsed, if canned)
2 cups shredded lettuce
1 cup corn (drained and
   rinsed, if canned)
Pico de Gallo (page 175),
   for topping (optional)
Avocado or guacamole,
   for topping (optional)
Salsa, for topping
   (optional)

To make the seasoning

1. In a small bowl, combine all the ingredients and stir well. Set aside.

To make the burritos

2. In a nonstick pan over high heat, bring the broth and water to a boil. Add the TVP and the seasoning and combine. Reduce the heat to low, cover the pan, and simmer, stirring frequently, for 5 minutes, or until the TVP has absorbed all the moisture and is soft.

(continued)

TVP Burritos (continued)

3. On a large plate, place 1 tortilla and top with one-quarter of the TVP mixture, rice, beans, lettuce, corn, and toppings (if using). Fold in the sides of the tortilla and roll it up. Repeat with the remaining tortillas and ingredients.

Per serving: Calories: 654; Total fat: 8g; Carbohydrates: 111g; Fiber: 24g; Protein: 34g; Calcium: 15%; Vitamin D: 0%; Vitamin B$_{12}$: 0%; Iron: 31%; Zinc: 12%

Prep Tip: Cook a large batch of brown rice (or quinoa, wild rice, or couscous) each week and store it in the refrigerator. It will be ready to go for recipes like this one, making meals easier and faster to prepare.

Recipe Tip: You can often find TVP in the health section of grocery stores, or more commonly in specialty stores and online.

Cream of Mushroom Soup

Prep time: 15 minutes, plus 1 hour
   to soak the cashews
Cook time: 25 minutes
SERVES 4

ENERGY BOOST **GLUTEN-FREE**

This warm, creamy soup is perfect on a cold day or when you're just looking for a comforting, flavorful meal. Enjoy this soup on its own or have it alongside a Veggie Rainbow Wrap (page 94), a big leafy green salad, or toasted bread.

1 cup cashews, soaked
   in hot water for at
   least 1 hour
1 cup water, divided
1 tablespoon freshly
   squeezed lemon juice
1 teaspoon white
   vinegar

¼ teaspoon pink
   Himalayan salt
¼ teaspoon
   Dijon mustard
1 small onion, diced
1 cup chopped
   fresh mushrooms
2 garlic cloves, minced

3 cups vegetable broth
2 tablespoons
   gluten-free flour
1 cup unsweetened
   plant-based milk
Freshly ground
   black pepper

1. In a food processor, combine the cashews, ¾ cup of water, the lemon juice, vinegar, salt, and mustard. Process until completely smooth and creamy. Set aside.

2. In a large nonstick pan over medium heat, sauté the onion, mushrooms, and garlic in the remaining ¼ cup of water for 3 to 5 minutes, or until the onion is soft.

3. Reduce the heat to medium low and add the broth and flour, whisking it together. Add the cashew cream base and milk and stir to combine well. Cover and simmer for 20 to 25 minutes, stirring occasionally, until the soup has thickened and the vegetables are soft. Serve immediately.

Per serving: Calories: 257; Total fat: 17g; Carbohydrates: 21g; Fiber: 3g; Protein: 8g; Calcium: 15%; Vitamin D: 11%; Vitamin B$_{12}$: 13%; Iron: 16%; Zinc: 15%

Storage Tip: This soup stores well in a reusable container in the refrigerator for up to 5 days. Reheat leftovers in a nonstick pot over medium heat, stirring frequently.

Mushroom Stroganoff

Prep time: 10 minutes

Cook time: 20 minutes

SERVES 4

STRENGTH BUILDER   GLUTEN-FREE   NUT-FREE

This creamy, savory noodle dish is a veganized comfort food favorite. In addition to the plant-based swaps, I've replaced the traditional egg noodles with rice noodles, which cook perfectly together with the sauce.

- 1 medium onion, chopped
- 1 garlic clove, minced
- 3¼ cups vegetable broth, divided
- 1 (350-gram) block firm tofu, cubed
- 3 cups chopped mushrooms
- 3 tablespoons gluten-free flour
- ⅛ teaspoon dried thyme
- 1 tablespoon Dijon mustard
- 1 tablespoon vegan Worcestershire sauce (check label for gluten-free)
- ½ teaspoon freshly ground black pepper
- ¼ teaspoon pink Himalayan salt
- ¼ teaspoon apple cider vinegar
- ¼ cup unsweetened plant-based milk
- 10 ounces uncooked rice noodles
- ½ cup water, plus up to ¼ cup more if needed

1. In a large nonstick pan over medium heat, sauté the onion and garlic in ¼ cup of broth for 5 minutes, or until soft. Add the tofu, mushrooms, and the remaining 3 cups of broth. Whisk in the flour and thyme. Stir in the mustard, Worcestershire sauce, pepper, salt, and vinegar. Bring to a boil, then reduce the heat to low.

2. Add the milk and rice noodles. Stir until the noodles are mixed well into the sauce, add the water, and cover the pan. Simmer, stirring frequently, for 10 minutes, or until the noodles are soft. If needed, add more water to soften the rice noodles.

3. Serve immediately, or store in a reusable container in the refrigerator for 5 days.

Per serving: Calories: 419; Total fat: 7g; Carbohydrates: 73g; Fiber: 4g; Protein: 18g; Calcium: 13%; Vitamin D: 12%; Vitamin B_{12}: <1%; Iron: 17%; Zinc: 2%

Recipe Tip: This dish goes great with a side of Cucumber Dill Salad (page 112).

Sesame Soba Noodles with Tempeh

Prep time: 10 minutes
Cook time: 20 minutes

SERVES 4

RECOVERY   NUT-FREE

Soba noodles are thin and look like spaghetti but are made from buckwheat, which is high in the minerals and antioxidants that can aid your recovery after strenuous activity. This delightful and easy-to-make dish can be eaten warm or cold.

For the sauce

6 tablespoons
    tahini paste
¼ cup water
4 tablespoons freshly
    squeezed lemon juice
4-inch fresh ginger
    root, minced
4 teaspoons apple
    cider vinegar
4 teaspoons
    maple syrup
4 teaspoons red
    pepper flakes

4 teaspoons low-sodium
    soy sauce (or
    tamari, which is a
    gluten-free option)
½ teaspoon pink
    Himalayan salt
½ teaspoon freshly
    ground black pepper

For the noodles

12 slices tempeh
2 tablespoons water
¼ teaspoon freshly
    ground black pepper

¼ teaspoon pink
    Himalayan salt
8 ounces cooked
    soba noodles
1 red bell
    pepper, chopped
1 carrot, chopped
1 cup snow peas
1 cup sliced mushrooms
Scallions, chopped, for
    topping (optional)
Sesame seeds, for
    topping (optional)

To make the sauce

1. In a bowl, combine all the ingredients and mix well.

(continued)

Sesame Soba Noodles with Tempeh (continued)

To make the noodles

2. In a large nonstick pan over medium heat, warm the tempeh with the water, pepper, and salt for 3 to 5 minutes, continuously flipping the tempeh. Add the sauce, noodles, bell pepper, carrot, snow peas, and mushrooms and stir together. Reduce the heat to medium, cover the pan with a lid, and cook, stirring frequently, for 10 to 15 minutes. Serve immediately, garnished with scallions and sesame seeds (if using), or store in a reusable container in the refrigerator for up to 5 days.

Per serving: Calories: 444; Total fat: 16g; Carbohydrates: 63g; Fiber: 6g; Protein: 19g; Calcium: 21%; Vitamin D: 3%; Vitamin B$_{12}$: <1%; Iron: 23%; Zinc: 17%

Substitution Tip: Try adding different vegetables, such as broccoli, spinach, or bok choy, to your soba noodles.

Sloppy Joes

Prep time: 10 minutes

Cook time: 15 minutes

SERVES 4

STRENGTH BUILDER **GLUTEN-FREE OPTION**

NUT-FREE

This sweet, savory, and smoky sandwich is a veganized classic. Traditionally, this sandwich includes ground beef, which I've replaced with chickpeas and lentils. These Sloppy Joes have plenty of protein and bold flavors without the animal ingredients, saturated fat, or cholesterol. They're really tasty, so it's completely worth it if you get a little messy!

1 cup cooked chickpeas (drained and rinsed, if canned)

½ cup ketchup

⅛ cup water, plus ¼ cup

1 tablespoon maple syrup

1 teaspoon vegan Worcestershire sauce (check label for gluten-free)

½ teaspoon garlic powder

¼ teaspoon pink Himalayan salt

⅛ teaspoon freshly ground black pepper

1 small yellow onion, diced

1 cup cooked lentils (drained and rinsed, if canned)

4 vegan gluten-free or whole wheat buns

1. In a bowl, roughly mash the chickpeas with a potato masher.

2. In a separate bowl, mix the ketchup, ⅛ cup of water, maple syrup, Worcestershire sauce, garlic powder, salt, and pepper. Set aside.

3. In a nonstick pan over medium heat, combine the onion and ¼ cup of water and cook for 3 minutes. Add the chickpeas and lentils and mix. Add the sauce and cook, covered, for 10 minutes, stirring frequently.

4. Serve immediately on the buns, or store in the refrigerator for up to 5 days.

Per serving: Calories: 321; Total fat: 3g; Carbohydrates: 63g; Fiber: 11g; Protein: 14g; Calcium: 4%; Vitamin D: 0%; Vitamin B$_{12}$: 0%; Iron: 22%; Zinc: 10%

Recipe Tip: Top these Sloppy Joes with Colorful Coleslaw (page 110).

Substitution Tip: Skip the buns and use the Sloppy Joes to top 4 baked potatoes.

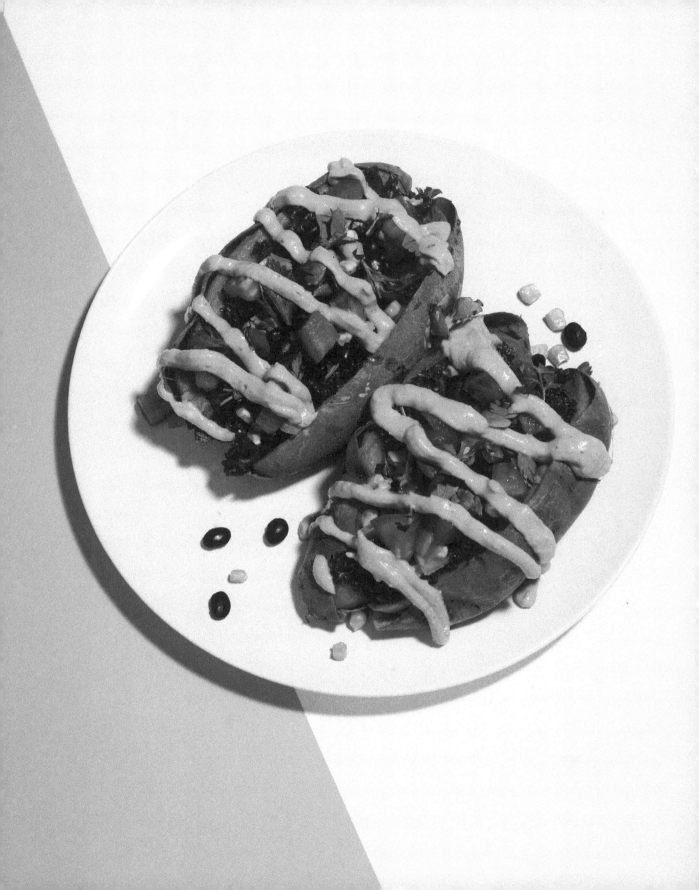

Snacks and Sides

Loaded Baked Sweet Potatoes, 122

Maple Crunch Granola

Prep time: 5 minutes

Cook time: 25 minutes

SERVES 4

Granola is an excellent snack that keeps you feeling full of sustained energy for a busy day, a hike, or training. This granola is packed with fiber, vitamins, minerals, omega-3 fatty acids, protein, and antioxidants. Enjoy it on its own or served with vegan unsweetened plain yogurt and fresh fruit.

2 cups rolled oats (check label for gluten-free)

1 cup maple syrup

¼ cup chopped walnuts

¼ cup chopped almonds

¼ cup chopped pecans

2 tablespoons sunflower seeds

2 tablespoons pumpkin seeds

1 tablespoon hemp seed

1 teaspoon vanilla extract

1. Preheat the oven to 350°F. Line a baking sheet with parchment paper or a silicone liner.

2. In a large bowl, stir together all the ingredients until thoroughly mixed.

3. Spread out the mixture on the prepared baking sheet and bake for 25 minutes, or until lightly browned. Stir the granola at the halfway mark to ensure an even bake. Remove from the oven and allow it to cool before serving.

Per serving: Calories: 553; Total fat: 21g; Carbohydrates: 85g; Fiber: 7g; Protein: 11g; Calcium: 9%; Vitamin D: 0%; Vitamin B$_{12}$: 2%; Iron: 23%; Zinc: 30%

Storage Tip: Store at room temperature in a sealed container for up to 10 days.

Substitution Tip: Try adding different nuts, seeds, and dried fruit to switch up the flavor.

Artichoke-Spinach Dip

Prep time: 15 minutes, plus 1 hour to soak the cashews
Cook time: 25 minutes
SERVES 6

ENERGY BOOST

GLUTEN-FREE

This creamy, nutrient-packed dip can be enjoyed with veggie sticks or whole-grain bread or crackers.

2 cups chopped cauliflower
3 garlic cloves, crushed
1 cup cashews, soaked in hot water for at least 1 hour
½ cup water
2 teaspoons Dijon mustard

2 teaspoons pink Himalayan salt
2 teaspoons freshly squeezed lemon juice
1½ teaspoons freshly ground black pepper
1½ teaspoons red pepper flakes
1 teaspoon white vinegar

1 (14-ounce) can artichoke hearts, drained and chopped
1 cup frozen spinach, thawed and strained
Parmesan Cheese (page 183), for topping (optional)

1. Preheat the oven to 350°F.
2. In a pot over medium-high heat, boil the cauliflower and garlic in water for 10 minutes, or until the garlic has softened. Remove from the heat, strain, and set aside to cool.
3. Once cooled, in a food processor, combine the cauliflower and garlic with the cashews, water, mustard, salt, lemon juice, black pepper, red pepper flakes, and vinegar. Blend until smooth.
4. Transfer the mixture to a large bowl and stir in the artichoke hearts and spinach.
5. Transfer the mixture to an 8-inch square casserole dish and bake for 15 minutes, or until lightly browned on the top and edges.

Per serving: Calories: 260; Total fat: 16g; Carbohydrates: 24g; Fiber: 6g; Protein: 10g; Calcium: 10%; Vitamin D: 0% Vitamin B$_{12}$: 0%; Iron: 18%; Zinc: 16%

Storage Tip: Serve hot or cold. Store in the refrigerator for up to 5 days.

Baked Onion Rings

Prep time: 5 minutes
Cook time: 10 minutes
SERVES 2

I love onion rings, but I've never really liked how greasy they can be, which is why I developed these delicious onion rings that are baked, not fried. These make a great snack on their own, or you can try them alongside Chickpea Burgers (page 136).

1 cup vegan
  bread crumbs
½ teaspoon paprika
¼ teaspoon
  garlic powder

¼ teaspoon freshly
  ground black pepper
¼ teaspoon pink
  Himalayan salt
¾ cup water

½ cup whole
  wheat flour
2 large yellow onions,
  cut into ½-inch rings

1. Preheat the oven to 400°F. Line a baking sheet with parchment paper or a silicone liner.

2. In a bowl, blend the bread crumbs, paprika, garlic powder, pepper, and salt.

3. In a separate bowl, blend the water and flour.

4. Dip each onion ring first into the wet ingredients and then into the dry ingredients, coating well. Place the coated onions rings on the prepared baking sheet and bake for 10 to 12 minutes, or until light brown. These are best enjoyed immediately after baking.

Per serving: Calories: 327; Total fat: 1g; Carbohydrates: 72g; Fiber: 8g; Protein: 10g; Calcium: 5%; Vitamin D: 0%; Vitamin B$_{12}$: 0%; Iron: 12%; Zinc: 2%

Recipe Tip: If your vegan bread crumbs are large, blend them in the food processor until they resemble a rough powder. They'll coat the onions better, and your onion rings will be crispier.

Lemon and Black Pepper Edamame

Prep time: 5 minutes
Cook time: 5 minutes
SERVES 2

STRENGTH BUILDER **GLUTEN-FREE** **NUT-FREE**

The distinctive tastes of fresh lemon and black pepper, balanced with a touch of salt, makes these poppable edamame a healthy and delightful snack you can eat with your hands.

Zest of 1 lemon

2 tablespoons freshly squeezed lemon juice

¼ teaspoon freshly ground black pepper

⅛ teaspoon pink Himalayan salt

2 cups edamame, unshelled

1. In a small bowl, combine the lemon zest, lemon juice, pepper, and salt.
2. Steam or boil the edamame for 5 minutes. Remove from the heat and place in a big bowl. Pour the lemon-pepper mixture over the edamame and toss until covered thoroughly. Enjoy warm or store in a reusable container in the refrigerator for up to 5 days.

Per serving: Calories: 366; Total fat: 15g; Carbohydrates: 29g; Fiber: 9g; Protein: 30g; Calcium: 30%; Vitamin D: 0%; Vitamin B$_{12}$: 0%; Iron: 31%; Zinc: <1%

Nutrition Tip: Edamame aren't just a protein powerhouse; they are also packed with calcium, iron, folate, manganese, potassium, fiber, and vitamins C, K, and E.

Cheesy Kale Chips

Prep time: 10 minutes
Cook time: 10 minutes

SERVES 4

GRAB AND GO   GLUTEN-FREE

This recipe might just be the epitome of healthy snacking. These flavorful kale chips are not only delicious, they're also loaded with antioxidants, beta-carotene, and vitamins K, C, and B_6. Plus, the fortified nutritional yeast is a great source of B_{12}. This snack is a superfood, and it's always a good idea to eat nutrient-dense foods such as kale as often as possible.

6 tablespoons
    Parmesan Cheese
    (page 183)

3 tablespoons freshly
    squeezed lemon juice
Pinch freshly ground
    black pepper

Pinch pink
    Himalayan salt
1 bunch kale, stems
    removed, chopped

1. Preheat the oven to 350°F. Line a baking sheet with parchment paper or a silicone liner.

2. In a bowl, mix the cheese, lemon juice, pepper, and salt. Rub the mixture into the kale.

3. Spread out the kale on the prepared baking sheet, making sure the pieces aren't overlapping. Bake for 8 to 12 minutes, or until crispy. Keep your eye on the chips while they're baking so they don't burn.

Per serving: Calories: 109; Total fat: 6g; Carbohydrates: 12g; Fiber: 4g; Protein: 5g; Calcium: 7%; Vitamin D: 0%; Vitamin B_{12}: 9%; Iron: 10%; Zinc: 8%

Recipe Tip: Wash the kale and dry it thoroughly before rubbing in the cheesy mixture.

Storage Tip: Store in a reusable container at room temperature for up to 5 days.

Chocolate Energy Balls

Prep time: 10 minutes

SERVES 3

GRAB AND GO **GLUTEN-FREE**

These are the perfect healthy snacks for athletes looking for quick fuel before training. They are made with energizing dates and almonds and have an appealing sweet and salty taste.

1 cup almonds

1½ tablespoons
 cocoa powder

⅛ teaspoon pink
 Himalayan salt

1 tablespoon
 maple syrup

10 Medjool dates, pitted
 and chopped

1. In a food processor, blend the almonds until they become a rough, grainy powder. Add the cocoa, salt, and maple syrup and blend well. Add the dates and blend until completely smooth.

2. Using your hands, shape the mixture into individual 1½-inch balls. Enjoy immediately or store in a reusable container at room temperature or in the refrigerator for up to 7 days.

Per serving (3 balls): Calories: 517; Total fat: 24g; Carbohydrates: 76g; Fiber: 12g; Protein: 12g; Calcium: 18%; Vitamin D: 0%; Vitamin B$_{12}$: 0%; Iron: 18%; Zinc: 16%

Prep Tip: If your dates are dry, soak them in warm water for 15 minutes to soften them before blending.

Colorful Coleslaw

Prep time: 10 minutes, plus 1 hour
   to soak the cashews

SERVES 4

This Colorful Coleslaw is the perfect addition to any barbecue. It's a simple, creamy, and healthy take on a summertime classic. Try it as a side with Chickpea Burgers (page 136).

½ cup cashews, soaked
   in hot water for at
   least 1 hour
2½ tablespoons white
   wine vinegar
¾ tablespoon
   coconut sugar

½ teaspoon pink
   Himalayan salt
¼ teaspoon freshly
   ground black pepper
2 cups shredded
   green cabbage

1 cup shredded
   purple cabbage
1 cup shredded carrots
1 cup shredded
   Brussels sprouts
½ cup water

1. In a food processor, combine the cashews, vinegar, coconut sugar, salt, water, and pepper. Blend well until creamy and smooth.

2. In a large bowl, combine the green cabbage, purple cabbage, carrots, and Brussels sprouts. Add the dressing and mix well. Serve immediately or store in a reusable container in the refrigerator for up to 5 days.

Per serving: Calories: 194; Total fat: 11g; Carbohydrates: 22g; Fiber: 5g; Protein: 6g; Calcium: 7%; Vitamin D: 0%; Vitamin B_{12}: 0%; Iron: 13%; Zinc: 11%

Nutrition Tip: Top the coleslaw with sunflower seeds for additional healthy essential fats, protein, copper, manganese, selenium, and vitamins B_3, B_6, B_9, and E.

Creamy Green Beans

Prep time: 5 minutes

Cook time: 15 minutes

SERVES 4

ENERGY BOOST **GLUTEN-FREE** **NUT-FREE**

Usually when vegetables are smothered in a rich sauce, the dish is heavy and high in fat, which defeats the purpose of eating fresh vegetables. Not this dish! These green beans swim in an easy-to-make, healthy, creamy sauce that doesn't skimp on flavor.

1 small yellow
  onion, diced

3 or 4 garlic
  cloves, minced

1 cup vegetable
  broth, divided

1 cup sliced mushrooms

1 cup unsweetened
  plant-based milk

2 tablespoons
  gluten-free flour

2 tablespoons
  B_{12}-fortified
  nutritional yeast

3 cups fresh
  green beans

Pink Himalayan salt

Freshly ground
  black pepper

1. In a large nonstick pan over medium heat, sauté the onion and garlic in ¼ cup of broth until the onion is soft. Add the mushrooms, milk, remaining ¾ cup of broth, flour, and nutritional yeast. Whisk until there are no clumps. Add the green beans, cover the pan with a lid, and cook on medium-low heat for 10 to 15 minutes, or until the beans are soft. Add salt and pepper to taste.

2. Serve immediately or store in a reusable container in the refrigerator for up to 5 days.

Per serving: Calories: 102; Total fat: 2g; Carbohydrates: 20g; Fiber: 7g; Protein: 6g; Calcium: 21%; Vitamin D: 13%; Vitamin B_{12}: 34%; Iron: 12%; Zinc: 9%

Substitution Tip: Try swapping out the green beans for spinach, green peas, or edamame.

Cucumber Dill Salad

Prep time: 5 minutes,
   plus 10 minutes to chill

SERVES 2

This Cucumber Dill Salad is super refreshing. Enjoy it on its own or as a side salad with virtually any main dish. It pairs especially well with a spicy meal, balancing the warm flavors with its cool freshness.

¼ cup water

3 tablespoons white
   wine vinegar

2 tablespoons chopped
   fresh dill

½ teaspoon
   coconut sugar

¼ teaspoon pink
   Himalayan salt

¼ teaspoon freshly
   ground black pepper

1 cucumber, cut into
   ¼-inch-thick rounds

1 red onion, thinly sliced

▶ In a medium bowl, combine the water, vinegar, dill, coconut sugar, salt, and pepper and mix well. Add the cucumber and red onion and stir to mix with the dressing. Chill in the refrigerator for 10 minutes before serving.

Per serving: Calories: 50; Total fat: <1g; Carbohydrates: 10g; Fiber: 2g; Protein: 2g; Calcium: 3%; Vitamin D: 0%; Vitamin B$_{12}$: 0%; Iron: 4%; Zinc: 3%

Recipe Tip: The longer you let the cucumbers and red onions marinate in the dressing, the more flavorful the salad will be. This stores well in a reusable container in the refrigerator for up to 5 days.

Loaded Apple Nachos

Prep time: 10 minutes

SERVES 4

Loaded with healthy carbs, potassium, minerals, and antioxidants, these nachos can be great fuel before training. They pair a sweet and sour Granny Smith apple with a delicious date sauce, vegan dark chocolate chips, pecans, and hemp seeds.

1 cup Medjool dates, pitted

½ cup unsweetened plant-based milk

1 teaspoon vanilla extract

⅛ teaspoon pink Himalayan salt

4 Granny Smith apples, cored and cut into ¼-inch slices

¼ cup pecans, chopped

2 tablespoons vegan dark chocolate chips

1 teaspoon hemp seeds

1. Blend the dates in a food processor until they resemble a paste. Add the milk, vanilla, and salt, and blend until smooth. Set aside.

2. On a plate, lay out 1 sliced apple (use 1 apple per serving on individual plates). Drizzle 1 tablespoon of the date sauce over the apple. Top with 1 tablespoon of pecans, ½ tablespoon of chocolate chips, and ¼ teaspoon of hemp seeds. Repeat with the remaining apples and toppings.

Per serving: Calories: 318; Total fat: 9g; Carbohydrates: 64g; Fiber: 9g; Protein: 3g; Calcium: 8%; Vitamin D: 3%; Vitamin B$_{12}$: 1%; Iron: 5%; Zinc: 4%

Storage Tip: Store the date sauce in a reusable container in the refrigerator for up to 5 days, until you're ready to assemble and eat the nachos.

Soft Pretzels

Prep time: 1 hour 15 minutes
Cook time: 25 minutes

GRAB AND GO **NUT-FREE**

SERVES 8

These are higher in protein than your average pretzel. I use whole wheat flour and vital wheat gluten to create a light, fluffy, soft pretzel that tastes great and is a fun on-the-go snack.

2¼ teaspoons active
    dry yeast
1 tablespoon sugar
1½ cups warm water

2½ cups whole
    wheat flour
¼ cup vital
    wheat gluten

10 cups water
⅔ cup baking soda
Pink Himalayan
    salt (optional)

1. Stir the yeast and sugar into the warm water and let it sit for 10 to 15 minutes.

2. In a large bowl, combine the flour and wheat gluten. Add the yeast mixture and mix well.

3. Knead the dough by hand for 5 minutes. Form the dough into a ball and place it in a clean bowl. Cover the bowl and let it sit for 50 to 60 minutes to allow the dough to rise.

4. Preheat the oven to 450°F. Line a baking sheet with parchment paper.

5. Remove the dough from the bowl and cut it into 8 equal pieces. Roll the pieces into ropes 15 to 18 inches long. Shape the ropes into pretzels.

6. Pour 10 cups of water into a pot. Set over high heat and add the baking soda. Bring to a boil and cook each pretzel, one at a time, for 30 to 45 seconds.

7. Place the pretzels on the prepared baking sheet. Bake for 12 to 14 minutes, or until lightly browned. Sprinkle with salt (if using). Enjoy warm or store in a reusable container at room temperature for 3 to 5 days.

Per serving: Calories: 158; Total fat: 1g; Carbohydrates: 31g; Fiber: 5g; Protein: 7g; Calcium: 3%; Vitamin D: 0%; Vitamin B$_{12}$: 0%; Iron: 11%; Zinc: <1%

Substitution Tip: For a sweet taste, try topping your pretzels with cinnamon and coconut sugar after they come out of the oven.

Nut Butter Protein Bites

Prep time: 10 minutes

MAKES 9 BITES

GRAB AND GO GLUTEN-FREE

These craveable and nutritious nut butter bites are a fan favorite. They don't last long at my house, so don't be surprised if you need to make a bigger batch.

½ cup almond or peanut butter

½ cup rolled oats (check label for gluten-free)

¼ cup ground chia seeds

3 tablespoons maple syrup

1 tablespoon ground flaxseed

1 tablespoon pumpkin seeds

1. Combine all the ingredients in a food processor and blend well, until very small bits of the seeds are still visible.

2. Using your hands, shape the mixture into small balls and enjoy immediately or store in a reusable container at room temperature or in the refrigerator for up to 10 days.

Per serving: Calories: 154; Total fat: 10g; Carbohydrates: 13g; Fiber: 4g; Protein: 6g; Calcium: 6%; Vitamin D: 0%; Vitamin B_{12}: 0%; Iron: 6%; Zinc: 5%

Prep Tip: These are perfect snacks to add to your meal prep. They're great before or after training, and anytime in between.

Classic Stuffing

Prep time: 10 minutes, or overnight
Cook time: 40 minutes

SERVES 6

My mom's stuffing has always been one of my absolute favorite dishes during the holidays, so I had to veganize it. The flavor and texture are as delicious as ever, and it's even better knowing that I don't have to deal with stuffing it into a turkey.

1½ (20-ounce) loaves whole wheat bread, broken into small pieces

2 cups vegetable broth
5 celery stalks, chopped
1 large yellow onion, chopped

3 tablespoons vegan poultry seasoning

1. Preheat the oven to 350°F.

2. In a large roasting pan, combine all the ingredients and stir together until everything is well mixed and the bread is evenly moistened. Cover the pan with aluminum foil and bake for 40 minutes.

3. You can serve this stuffing immediately or store in a reusable container in the refrigerator.

Per serving: Calories: 608; Total fat: 11g; Carbohydrates: 113g; Fiber: 14g; Protein: 18g; Calcium: 71%; Vitamin D: 0%; Vitamin B$_{12}$: 0%; Iron: 12%; Zinc: 24%

Recipe Tip: The recipe works best if you break up the bread the night before you cook the dish, keeping the pieces uncovered in the pan to allow the bread to harden.

Potato Salad

Prep time: 10 minutes
Cook time: 15 minutes
SERVES 4

ENERGY BOOST   **GLUTEN-FREE**

A summer favorite made delicious and vegan. There's quite a bit of mayonnaise in potato salads, but since we're using my Mighty Mayo, this recipe delivers the classic creamy taste you love, without the usual heavy oil base.

6 medium potatoes, cubed and boiled

¾ cup Mighty Mayo (page 182)

2 celery stalks, diced

2 or 3 scallions, chopped

2 dill pickles, chopped

2 tablespoons yellow mustard

Freshly ground black pepper

Pink Himalayan salt

Ground paprika (optional)

1. Cook the potatoes in boiling water for 15 minutes, or until tender but still a little firm. Drain and rinse the potatoes in cool water.

2. In a bowl, combine the potatoes, mayo, celery, scallions, pickles, and mustard and season with pepper and salt to taste. Mix until thoroughly coated. Sprinkle with paprika (if using). Enjoy immediately or store in a reusable container in the refrigerator for up to 5 days.

Per serving: Calories: 375; Total fat: 13g; Carbohydrates: 63g; Fiber: 9g; Protein: 9g; Calcium: 10%; Vitamin D: 3%; Vitamin B_{12}: 0%; Iron: 24%; Zinc: 16%

Nutrition Tip: Try leaving the skin on the potatoes to benefit from the added fiber, vitamins, and minerals.

Garlic Cauliflower Mashed Potatoes

Prep time: 10 minutes
Cook time: 20 minutes
SERVES 4

ENERGY BOOST   **GLUTEN-FREE**   **NUT-FREE**

Mashed potatoes are one of my favorite side dishes. Well, anything with potatoes is usually going to be a hit with me. Here, I've combined cauliflower with the potatoes to boost the nutritional variety, and I added sautéed garlic for a distinctive flavor that makes this side dish a home run for potato and garlic lovers alike.

5 medium yellow
  potatoes, chopped
¾ cup unsweetened
  plant-based milk

Pink Himalayan salt
Freshly ground
  black pepper
½ medium cauliflower

6 garlic cloves, minced
¼ cup vegetable broth

1. In a big pot over medium-high heat, boil the potatoes for 15 minutes, or until soft. When cooked, drain and return the potatoes to the pot. Mash the potatoes while beating in the milk. Season with salt and pepper.

2. In a vegetable steamer, steam the cauliflower for 10 minutes. Transfer it to a food processor and blend until roughly smooth.

3. In a nonstick pan over medium heat, sauté the garlic in the broth for 5 minutes, or until soft.

4. Transfer the cauliflower and garlic to the big pot with the mashed potatoes. Combine by using a potato masher or stirring well. Serve warm. This stores well in a reusable container in the refrigerator for up to 5 days.

Per serving: Calories: 169; Total fat: 1g; Carbohydrates: 38g; Fiber: 5g; Protein: 6g; Calcium: 14%; Vitamin D: 5%; Vitamin B$_{12}$: 0%; Iron: 11%; Zinc: 4%

Recipe Tip: Try this as a side with Meat-Free Loaf (page 154).

Spicy Thai-Inspired Vegetables

Prep time: 10 minutes
Cook time: 10 minutes
SERVES 2

ENERGY BOOST **GLUTEN-FREE OPTION**

NUT-FREE

This delightful combination of mild spicy and sweet flavors with steamed mixed vegetables goes well with brown rice, wild rice, quinoa, or rice noodles.

5 broccoli florets

5 baby bok choy

½ red bell pepper

½ cup edamame, shelled

¼ cup rice vinegar

¼ cup water, plus 1 tablespoon

3 garlic cloves, minced

4 teaspoons red pepper flakes

½ tablespoon low-sodium soy sauce (or tamari, which is a gluten-free option)

1 tablespoon maple syrup

¼ teaspoon garlic powder

1 teaspoon gluten-free flour

1. Steam the broccoli, bok choy, bell pepper, and edamame for 10 minutes, or until tender.

2. In a small saucepan, combine the vinegar, ¼ cup of water, garlic, red pepper flakes, soy sauce, maple syrup, and garlic powder.

3. In a bowl, mix the flour with the remaining 1 tablespoon of water, then add the slurry to the saucepan. Stir the sauce until it thickens.

4. Remove the vegetables from the steamer and transfer to a large bowl. Pour the sauce over the vegetables and mix until thoroughly covered. Serve immediately or store in a reusable container in the refrigerator for up to 5 days.

Per serving: Calories: 151; Total fat: 1g; Carbohydrates: 26g; Fiber: 2g; Protein: 17g; Calcium: 7%; Vitamin D: 0%; Vitamin B$_{12}$: 0%; Iron: 7%; Zinc: 4%

Nutrition Tip: To get more protein, add tofu or tempeh.

Slow Cooker Baked Beans

Prep time: 5 minutes,
    plus overnight to soak the beans
Cook time: 6 to 8 hours

SERVES 4

STRENGTH BUILDER   GLUTEN-FREE

NUT-FREE

This recipe takes a little preparation because you'll be soaking the beans overnight, but you can leave everything in the slow cooker the next morning and dinner will be ready when you get home. This homemade version of sweet and smoky baked beans is far tastier than what you get with store-bought cans, and it's budget-friendly, too.

1½ cups water

1 cup tomato sauce

⅓ cup molasses

¼ cup brown sugar

1 tablespoon apple
    cider vinegar

1 tablespoon mustard

½ teaspoon pink
    Himalayan salt

½ teaspoon freshly
    ground black pepper

2 cups dried navy beans,
    soaked overnight
    and drained

1 medium yellow
    onion, chopped

1. In a mixing bowl, combine the water, tomato sauce, molasses, brown sugar, vinegar, mustard, salt, and pepper.

2. In a slow cooker, combine the beans, onion, and the sauce. Set the slow cooker for 6 to 8 hours on Low, until the beans are tender.

3. Enjoy warm or store in a reusable container in the refrigerator for up to 7 days.

Per serving: Calories: 325; Total fat: <1g; Carbohydrates: 82g; Fiber: 20g; Protein: 17g; Calcium: 20%; Vitamin D: 0%; Vitamin B$_{12}$: 0%; Iron: 42%; Zinc: 2%

Recipe Tip: Slow cookers vary, so if your baked beans look a little dry, stir in an additional ½ cup of water at a time, as needed.

Scalloped Potatoes

Prep time: 10 minutes,
   plus 1 hour to soak the cashews
Cook time: 40 minutes
SERVES 4

RECOVERY   GLUTEN-FREE

These rich and creamy scalloped potatoes are almost a meal in themselves. Potatoes smothered in a cheesy-flavored, cashew-based sauce makes this dish a satisfying comfort food that's still healthy and nutrient-packed. It's the best of both worlds.

1 cup cashews, soaked
   in hot water for at
   least 1 hour
¾ cup vegetable broth
½ cup unsweetened
   plant-based milk

2 tablespoons
   B_{12}-fortified
   nutritional yeast
2 teaspoons pink
   Himalayan salt
1 teaspoon paprika

1 teaspoon freshly
   ground black pepper
½ teaspoon
   onion powder
5 small yellow
   potatoes, peeled and
   thinly sliced

1. Preheat the oven to 400°F.

2. In a food processor, combine the cashews and broth and blend until completely smooth. Add the milk, nutritional yeast, salt, paprika, pepper, and onion powder. Blend until mixed well.

3. In an 8-inch square glass casserole dish, spread a thin layer of sauce. Lay half the potatoes on top and pour half of the remaining sauce evenly over them. Layer the rest of the potatoes on top, and cover with the rest of the sauce.

4. Cover with aluminum foil and cook for 30 minutes. Uncover and cook for another 10 minutes. Serve warm or store in a reusable container in the refrigerator for up to 7 days.

Per serving: Calories: 320; Total fat: 16g; Carbohydrates: 37g; Fiber: 5g; Protein: 11g; Calcium: 11%; Vitamin D: 3%; Vitamin B_{12}: 25%; Iron: 39%; Zinc: 17%

Recipe Tip: This goes well on the side with Meat-Free Loaf (page 154) or Air-Fried Chicken-Style Seitan (page 127).

Loaded Baked Sweet Potatoes

Prep time: 5 minutes
Cook time: 50 minutes
SERVES 2

PRE-GAME **GLUTEN-FREE** **NUT-FREE**

Loaded Baked Sweet Potatoes are the side dish that eats like a meal. They're packed with wholesome ingredients that are perfect for athletes looking for a nutritious and tasty meal to fuel their active lifestyle. They also go well with Maple-Garlic Air-Fried Tofu (page 143) or Air-Fried Chicken-Style Seitan (page 127).

2 sweet potatoes
2 cups fresh kale
1 cup cooked black beans (drained and rinsed, if canned)

½ cup corn, frozen or canned
½ small red onion, diced
¼ cup vegetable broth or water

¾ cup chopped fresh tomatoes
Fresh cilantro, chopped
Creamy Avocado Dressing (page 177)

1. Preheat the oven to 400°F.

2. Poke several holes all over the sweet potatoes with a fork. Bake on a baking sheet for 50 minutes, or until tender.

3. While the potatoes are cooking, warm the kale, beans, corn, and onion in a nonstick pan over medium heat with the broth, covered with a lid but stirring frequently, for 10 minutes, or until the onion has softened.

4. Remove the potatoes from the oven, cut down the center of each, and push the ends toward each other to open up the potato. Place the vegetable mixture on top. Add the tomatoes and cilantro, and drizzle with the dressing.

Per serving: Calories: 685; Total fat: 4g; Carbohydrates: 143g; Fiber: 32g; Protein: 29g; Calcium: 31%; Vitamin D: 0%; Vitamin B$_{12}$: 0%; Iron: 48%; Zinc: 25%

Storage Tip: Store the ingredients separately in reusable containers in the refrigerator for up to 5 days, and top the sweet potato when ready to eat.

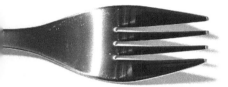
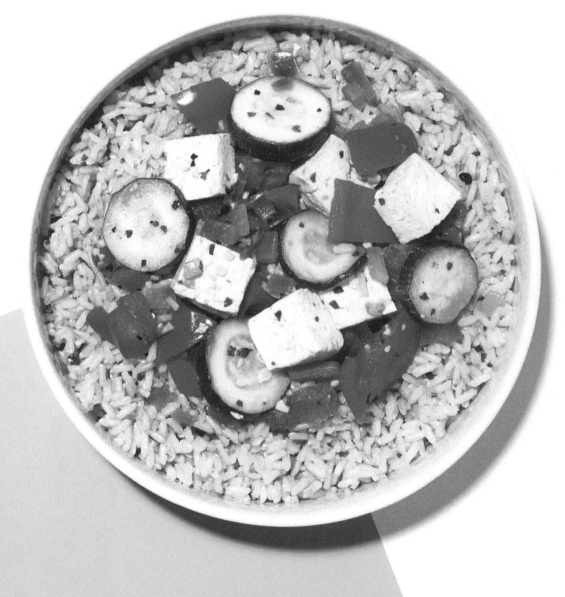

Dinner

Turmeric Italian Tofu and Rice, 150

5-Bean Chili

Prep time: 10 minutes

Cook time: 1 hour

SERVES 8

RECOVERY **GLUTEN-FREE** **NUT-FREE**

Chili is one of the tastiest ways to leverage the goodness of heart-healthy, protein-packed beans. This dish is a crowd-pleaser, perfect for potlucks and family gatherings.

2 (26- to 28-ounce) cans diced tomatoes

1 (19-ounce) can red kidney beans, drained and rinsed

1 (19-ounce) can white kidney beans, drained and rinsed

1 (19-ounce) can chickpeas, drained and rinsed

1 (19-ounce) can black beans, drained and rinsed

1 (19-ounce) can pinto beans, drained and rinsed

2½ cups fresh mushrooms, sliced

1 medium red bell pepper, chopped

1 large yellow onion, chopped

1 cup corn, canned or frozen

1½ tablespoons chili powder

1 teaspoon ground cumin

½ teaspoon freshly ground black pepper

½ teaspoon pink Himalayan salt

¼ teaspoon cayenne pepper

¼ teaspoon garlic powder

1. Combine all the ingredients in a large pot over medium heat. Cover the pot with a lid and cook, stirring occasionally, for 45 to 60 minutes.

2. Serve as is, or on a bed of brown rice, quinoa, or with a fresh avocado. If you have leftovers or you're doing meal prep, store in reusable containers in the refrigerator for up to 5 days or freeze for up to 2 months.

Per serving: Calories: 756; Total fat: 5g; Carbohydrates: 139g; Fiber: 44g; Protein: 41g; Calcium: 26%; Vitamin D: 8%; Vitamin B$_{12}$: <1%; Iron: 58%; Zinc: 35%

Recipe Tip: To make the chili thicker, cook uncovered for another 15 to 20 minutes.

Air-Fried Chicken-Style Seitan

Prep time: 20 minutes

Cook time: 1 hour

SERVES 2

`STRENGTH BUILDER`   `NUT-FREE`

Seitan is a great meat alternative that's high in protein but low in fat and carbohydrates. It's also less expensive than many store-bought plant-based meats, so it's an excellent option for vegans on a budget. Try adding Bold Barbecue Sauce (page 84) to the air fryer while this cooks.

1 cup vital wheat gluten

2 tablespoons whole wheat flour

1 teaspoon vegan poultry seasoning

1 tablespoon B_{12}-fortified nutritional yeast

1 teaspoon onion powder

1 teaspoon garlic powder

¼ teaspoon pink Himalayan salt

Pinch freshly ground black pepper

1 tablespoon aquafaba (the liquid from a can of chickpeas)

6¾ cups water, divided

1 vegan chick'n bouillon cube

1. In a large bowl, mix the gluten, flour, poultry seasoning, nutritional yeast, onion powder, garlic powder, salt, and pepper. Stir in the aquafaba and ¾ cup of water.

2. Knead the seitan dough together until the ingredients are mixed well. Transfer to a cutting board, roll out, and cut into 1-by-2-inch strips.

3. In a large pot over high heat, bring the remaining 6 cups of water and the bouillon cube to a boil. Reduce the heat to medium low. Add the seitan strips and simmer for 30 minutes. Drain the broth from the seitan pieces when ready to transfer to the air fryer.

4. Put the seitan strips in the air fryer and cook for 20 to 30 minutes, or until golden brown. Serve immediately or store in a sealed container for up to 7 days.

(continued)

Air-Fried Chicken-Style Seitan

(continued)

Per serving: Calories: 273; Total fat: 2g; Carbohydrates: 19g; Fiber: 3g; Protein: 48g; Calcium: 10%; Vitamin D: 0%; Vitamin B$_{12}$: 25%; Iron: 22%; Zinc: 8%

Prep Tip: Add this high-protein option to your meal prep for the week. Seitan is incredibly versatile; it goes well with everything from salads to veggies to potatoes.

Substitution Tip: This recipe uses an air fryer, but if you don't have one, you can bake the seitan in the oven at 350°F on a baking sheet lined with parchment paper or a silicone liner for 20 to 30 minutes, or until the edges are browned. The results won't be exactly the same as the air-fried version, but the dish will still turn out well.

Asparagus and Edamame Risotto

Prep time: 15 minutes
Cook time: 35 minutes

SERVES 2

ENERGY BOOST **GLUTEN-FREE** **NUT-FREE**

This risotto tastes rich and creamy without the fat. It's comfort food for those looking for a hearty meal without that uncomfortably stuffed feeling. One of the great benefits of asparagus is its ability to reduce bloating and water retention. This dish stores well in the refrigerator for up to 5 days, but I doubt it will last that long before you finish it.

12 asparagus spears

1 small onion, diced

3 garlic cloves, minced

¾ cup water, divided

3 cups vegetable broth

1 cup uncooked
   arborio rice

1 cup edamame, shelled

1 red bell
   pepper, chopped

1 tablespoon freshly
   squeezed lemon juice

1 tablespoon apple
   cider vinegar

¾ teaspoon freshly
   ground black pepper

½ teaspoon pink
   Himalayan salt

⅛ teaspoon
   garlic powder

⅛ teaspoon
   onion powder

1 cup unsweetened
   plant-based milk

1. In a vegetable steamer, cook the asparagus for 5 minutes.

2. In a large nonstick pan over medium-high heat, sauté the onion and garlic in ¼ cup of water for 5 minutes, or until soft. Reduce the heat to medium low, and add the asparagus, broth, rice, edamame, bell pepper, lemon juice, vinegar, pepper, salt, garlic powder, and onion powder and mix well. Cook for 15 minutes.

(continued)

Asparagus and Edamame Risotto (continued)

3. Add the milk and remaining ½ cup of water and stir frequently to blend. The sauce will begin to thicken. Continue to cook for 10 minutes.

4. Reduce the heat to low and simmer, covered, for about 5 minutes, or until the rice is tender. (You can add small amounts of water to continue cooking the rice, if needed.)

Per serving: Calories: 548; Total fat: 5g; Carbohydrates: 103g; Fiber: 9g; Protein: 23g; Calcium: 38%; Vitamin D: 15%; Vitamin B$_{12}$: 25%; Iron: 21%; Zinc: 6%

Nutrition Tip: Asparagus is a great source of fiber, folate, and vitamins K, A, C, and E. The vitamin C helps the body absorb nonheme (plant-based) iron.

Baked Falafel

Prep time: 30 minutes, plus overnight to
 soak the chickpeas
Cook time: 25 minutes

SERVES 3

I absolutely love falafel but have always hated how greasy it can be. This baked falafel solves that issue without losing flavor. It goes perfectly with Tabbouleh (page 91).

1 cup dried chickpeas

⅓ cup chopped
 fresh parsley

⅓ cup chopped
 fresh cilantro (most
 stems removed)

1 small red onion

2 tablespoons freshly
 squeezed lemon juice

1 teaspoon ground
 coriander

3 garlic cloves

½ teaspoon
 ground cumin

¼ teaspoon freshly
 ground black pepper

¼ teaspoon pink
 Himalayan salt

1. Soak the chickpeas in water overnight. Or, for a quicker option, bring water to a boil on the stove and add the chickpeas. Cover and reduce the heat to a simmer. Cook for 20 minutes, turn off the stove, and let it sit for 10 minutes. Drain and proceed with the recipe.

2. Preheat the oven to 400°F. Line a baking sheet with parchment paper or a silicone liner.

3. Combine all the ingredients in a food processor and blend until well mixed but some small bits remain. It should not be mushy.

4. Hand roll the mixture into 2-inch balls and place them on the prepared baking sheet. Cook for 25 to 30 minutes, or until lightly browned, rotating the balls at around the 15-minute mark.

Per serving (4 balls): Calories: 290; Total fat: 5g; Carbohydrates: 50g; Fiber: 14g; Protein: 16g; Calcium: 3%; Vitamin D: 0%; Vitamin B$_{12}$: 0%; Iron: 6%; Zinc: 2%

Baked Spaghetti Squash

Prep time: 5 minutes
Cook time: 40 minutes
SERVES 4

Want something light and fresh? Look no further. This simple dish is made with minimal ingredients. Spaghetti squash is often a great substitution for pasta, but it's also a legitimately delicious option on its own merits.

1 spaghetti squash
6 Roma tomatoes, chopped
½ small yellow onion, finely chopped
4 garlic cloves, minced
1 teaspoon dried basil

1 teaspoon red pepper flakes
1 teaspoon Italian seasoning
¼ teaspoon pink Himalayan salt
⅛ teaspoon freshly ground black pepper

1 cup sliced fresh mushrooms
2 cups fresh baby spinach
Parmesan Cheese (page 183), for topping (optional)

1. Preheat the oven to 400°F. Line a baking sheet with parchment paper or a silicone liner.

2. Cut the squash in half lengthwise. Place the squash halves cut-side down on the prepared baking sheet. Poke holes all over the skin with a fork.

3. Bake for 40 minutes. If you can't easily shred the insides of the squash with a fork, keep baking and check every 5 to 10 minutes.

4. While the squash is baking, in a medium nonstick pan over medium-high heat, combine the tomatoes, onion, garlic, basil, red pepper flakes, Italian seasoning, salt, and black pepper. Cook, stirring frequently, for 5 to 10 minutes, or until the tomatoes start to blend with the onion and garlic.

5. Use a fork to fluff up and remove the spaghetti strands from the skins. Transfer the strands to a bowl.

6. Add the mushrooms and spinach and cover. Reduce the heat to medium low and simmer for about 10 minutes, or until all the ingredients are fully cooked.

7. Add the sauce to the bowl of spaghetti squash and toss to combine. Sprinkle with Parmesan cheese (if using). Enjoy hot.

Per serving: Calories: 163; Total fat: 3g; Carbohydrates: 35g; Fiber: 7g; Protein: 6g; Calcium: 15%; Vitamin D: 4%; Vitamin B_{12}: <1%; Iron: 17%; Zinc: 5%

Nutrition Tip: Spaghetti squash is packed with vitamins, minerals, and antioxidants. This versatile winter vegetable is a good source of vitamin C, manganese, vitamin B_6, niacin, and potassium.

Storage Tip: This dish stores well in the refrigerator for up to 3 days.

Cabbage Rolls

Prep time: 20 minutes

Cook time: 1 hour 15 minutes

MAKES 8 TO 12 ROLLS

ENERGY BOOST   **GLUTEN-FREE**   **NUT-FREE**

These plant-powered cabbage rolls are a delicious low-fat, protein-rich meal that's satisfying and filling. This recipe takes a little preparation to pull together, but it's well worth it. To make the rolling easier, cut away any thick stems on the cabbage.

1 medium cabbage, whole, with core removed

1 medium yellow onion, chopped

3 garlic cloves, minced

¾ cup vegetable broth, divided

1 (19-ounce) can lentils, drained and rinsed

2 cups cooked brown rice

1 cup chopped fresh mushrooms

1 teaspoon dried basil

¼ teaspoon freshly ground black pepper

⅛ teaspoon pink Himalayan salt

3 cups tomato sauce

1. Preheat the oven to 350°F.

2. In a large stockpot over medium-high heat, boil the cabbage for about 15 minutes, or until the leaves are soft.

3. While the cabbage is cooking, in a large nonstick pan over medium heat, sauté the onion and garlic in ¼ cup of broth for 5 minutes. Add the lentils, rice, mushrooms, remaining ½ cup of broth, basil, pepper, and salt. Mix well and cover. Reduce the heat to low and cook, stirring occasionally, for 10 minutes.

4. Separate the cabbage leaves from the head. Place 2 to 3 tablespoons of the mixture into a cabbage leaf and roll it up like a little burrito. The mixture should make 8 to 12 rolls.

5. Spread a thin layer of tomato sauce on the bottom of a 9-by-13-inch glass pan. Lay the rolls on top and pour the remaining tomato sauce over the rolls. Cover the pan with aluminum foil and cook for 45 to 60 minutes, or until the rice is soft.

6. Enjoy immediately or store in a reusable container in the refrigerator for up to 5 days.

Per serving (3 rolls): Calories: 361; Total fat: 3g; Carbohydrates: 73g; Fiber: 19g; Protein: 18g; Calcium: 17%; Vitamin D: 3%; Vitamin B$_{12}$: <1%; Iron: 40%; Zinc: 15%

Substitution Tip: Boost the protein, magnesium, iron, and folate by swapping out the brown rice for quinoa.

Chickpea Burgers

Prep time: 5 minutes

Cook time: 10 minutes

SERVES 2

STRENGTH BUILDER

GLUTEN-FREE OPTION **NUT-FREE**

Some burgers have a bad rep because they are processed, but these change the game. They are easy to make, with just a few simple ingredients. Chickpea Burgers go great with a side of Colorful Coleslaw (page 110) and some Baked Onion Rings (page 106).

1 (19-ounce) can chickpeas, drained

½ cup vegan bread crumbs

⅛ cup aquafaba (the liquid from a can of chickpeas)

2 tablespoons chickpea flour

1 tablespoon low-sodium soy sauce (or tamari, which is a gluten-free option)

⅛ teaspoon pink Himalayan salt

⅛ teaspoon freshly ground black pepper

1. In a food processor, combine all the ingredients and pulse until roughly blended.

2. Using your hands, form the mixture into 2 patties.

3. In a nonstick pan over medium heat, cook the patties on each side for 5 minutes, or until lightly browned.

4. Serve on a whole-grain bun or lettuce wrap with your favorite condiments.

Per serving: Calories: 396; Total fat: 3g; Carbohydrates: 76g; Fiber: 12g; Protein: 16g; Calcium: 8%; Vitamin D: 0%; Vitamin B_{12}: 0%; Iron: 21%; Zinc: 17%

Nutrition Tip: Chickpea flour is an all-star vegan staple. It's high in protein, gluten-free, and loaded with vitamins, minerals, and antioxidants.

Gyro Pita with Tzatziki Sauce

Prep time: 10 minutes
Cook time: 15 minutes
SERVES 4

Ready for a delicious mix of fresh, cooling flavors? This gyro is a lighter, healthier version of its traditional counterpart. The taste of cucumber perfectly balances with the herbs and the fresh toppings here.

4 whole wheat pitas

For the tofu

2 tablespoons freshly
   squeezed lemon juice
1½ tablespoons
   dried oregano
1 tablespoon dried basil
1 tablespoon dried dill
1 tablespoon
   onion powder
1 tablespoon
   garlic powder
¼ teaspoon
   dried rosemary

⅛ teaspoon pink
   Himalayan salt
¼ teaspoon freshly
   ground black pepper
1 (350-gram) block firm
   tofu, cubed
½ cup vegetable broth

For the tzatziki sauce

1 cucumber,
   finely chopped
1 cup cashews
¼ cup unsweetened
   plant-based milk

3 garlic cloves
1½ tablespoons
   dried dill
1 tablespoon freshly
   squeezed lemon juice
2 teaspoons
   white vinegar

Toppings

1 large tomato, diced
2 cups chopped
   romaine lettuce
1 small red onion,
   thinly sliced

To make the tofu

1. In a medium bowl, combine the lemon juice, oregano, basil, dill, onion powder, garlic powder, rosemary, salt, and pepper.

2. In a medium nonstick pan over medium heat, cook the tofu, broth, and spiced lemon juice mixture, covered, for 10 to 15 minutes, stirring frequently.

(continued)

Gyro Pita with Tzatziki Sauce (continued)

To make the tzatziki sauce

3. In a food processor, combine all the ingredients and blend until smooth.

4. Serve the tofu in the pitas, topped with the tomato, lettuce, onion, and tzatziki sauce.

Per serving: Calories: 531; Total fat: 23g; Carbohydrates: 65g; Fiber: 11g; Protein: 25g; Calcium: 25%; Vitamin D: 2%; Vitamin B$_{12}$: 3%; Iron: 50%; Zinc: 24%

Storage Tip: Store the tofu and tzatziki sauce separately in the refrigerator for up to 5 days. Prepare the wraps when you're ready to eat.

Substitution Tip: For a gluten-free option, swap out the whole wheat pita for a romaine lettuce wrap, or serve over a bed of brown rice.

Curry Chickpeas and Potatoes

Prep time: 10 minutes
Cook time: 40 minutes

RECOVERY **GLUTEN-FREE** **NUT-FREE**

SERVES 3

This hearty, warm, and flavorful meal is comfort food at its best. To complement the bold spicy flavor, try adding some freshly cut cold cucumber slices or tomatoes on top. It stores well in the refrigerator for up to 5 days, making it great for meal prep.

1 medium
  onion, minced

3 garlic cloves, minced

2 tablespoons
  plant-based milk

2 teaspoons
  curry powder

¼ teaspoon
  cayenne pepper

½ teaspoon turmeric

½ teaspoon freshly
  ground black pepper

¼ teaspoon pink
  Himalayan salt

1⅓ cups water, divided

2 cups cooked
  chickpeas, or
  1 (19-ounce) can

2 medium ripe
  tomatoes, chopped

2 small yellow potatoes,
  chopped into
  small chunks

Juice of ½ lemon

1. In a medium nonstick pot over medium-high heat, sauté the onion, garlic, milk, curry powder, cayenne pepper, turmeric, black pepper, and salt in ⅓ cup of water, adding the water just a little at a time. The consistency will be thick. Add the remaining 1 cup of water, chickpeas, tomatoes, and potatoes. Stir until fully mixed, cover, reduce the heat to medium low, and simmer for 15 minutes, stirring frequently.

2. After 15 minutes, stir in the lemon juice and cover the pot. Simmer for another 15 minutes, or until the potatoes are soft. Uncover and cook for another 10 minutes, stirring occasionally.

3. Enjoy over a bed of steamed brown rice.

Per serving: Calories: 311; Total fat: 3g; Carbohydrates: 64g; Fiber: 11g; Protein: 12g; Calcium: 11%; Vitamin D: 1%; Vitamin B$_{12}$: 2%; Iron: 22%; Zinc: 15%

Curry Noodle Vegetable Soup

Prep time: 10 minutes
Cook time: 35 minutes
SERVES 4

This cozy curry noodle soup, with bold flavors and a nice golden color, is sure to keep you warm on a cold day. It will also satisfy all your noodle cravings.

½ onion, chopped

3 garlic cloves, minced

1-inch fresh ginger root, peeled and minced

4 cups vegetable broth, divided

2 cups unsweetened plant-based milk

½ (350-gram) block firm tofu, cubed

1 cup snap peas

1 cup bean sprouts

1 cup chopped mushrooms

1 tablespoon curry paste

1 teaspoon curry powder

1 teaspoon turmeric

1 teaspoon freshly ground black pepper

2 ounces wide rice noodles

1. In a large nonstick pot over medium heat, sauté the onion, garlic, and ginger in ¼ cup of broth until softened. Add the milk, the rest of the broth, tofu, snap peas, bean sprouts, mushrooms, curry paste, curry powder, turmeric, and pepper. Cover, reduce the heat to medium low, and continue to cook for 25 to 30 minutes, stirring occasionally. When all the vegetables are soft and the ingredients have cooked together, add the noodles, stir, cover, and cook for another 5 minutes, or until the noodles are soft.

2. Serve immediately or store in the refrigerator for up to 3 days.

Per serving: Calories: 161; Total fat: 4g; Carbohydrates: 24g; Fiber: 5g; Protein: 9g; Calcium: 30%; Vitamin D: 16%; Vitamin B_{12}: <1%; Iron: 14%; Zinc: 1%

Nutrition Tip: Curry powder contains an abundance of antioxidants and can help reduce oxidative stress in the body. Eat this distinctive and flavorful spice with black pepper to boost its direct absorption into the bloodstream.

Lentil Potato Soup

RECOVERY **GLUTEN-FREE** **NUT-FREE**

SERVES 4

Lentils and potatoes are two vegan staples that go great together. This soup is loaded with protein and healthy carbs, making it a nutritious—and delicious—meal any time.

2 medium
  onions, chopped

3 garlic cloves, chopped

4 cups water, divided

3 small potatoes,
  chopped

1 cup dried brown lentils

3 cups chopped kale

4 celery stalks, chopped

3 medium
  carrots, chopped

1 teaspoon turmeric

½ teaspoon freshly
  ground black pepper

½ teaspoon pink
  Himalayan salt

1. In a large nonstick pot over medium-high heat, sauté the onions and garlic in ¼ cup of water until softened.

2. Add the remaining 3¾ cups of water, the potatoes, lentils, kale, celery, carrots, turmeric, pepper, and salt and stir well. Reduce the heat to medium low, cover, and simmer for 40 minutes, or until the potatoes are soft.

Per serving: Calories: 332; Total fat: 1g; Carbohydrates: 66g; Fiber: 19g; Protein: 19g; Calcium: 17%; Vitamin D: 0%; Vitamin B_{12}: 0%; Iron: 42%; Zinc: 18%

Storage Tip: This stores well in the refrigerator for 5 to 7 days or in the freezer for 2 months.

Mushroom Barley Soup

Prep time: 10 minutes

Cook time: 40 minutes

SERVES 4

If you're looking for a hearty, filling soup that will warm you up and satisfy your hunger, this one's for you. Packed with pot barley and vegetables, it's a delicious and healthy way to fuel your active day.

2 small onions, chopped

3 garlic cloves, chopped

4 cups vegetable stock, divided

2 cups chopped white mushrooms

1 cup chopped baby portobello mushrooms

½ cup uncooked pot barley

1 carrot, finely chopped

1 celery stalk, finely chopped

1 vegan beef bouillon cube, or 1 tablespoon vegan gravy powder mixed with ½ cup cold water

1 teaspoon low-sodium soy sauce (or tamari, which is a gluten-free option)

¼ teaspoon freshly ground black pepper

¼ teaspoon pink Himalayan salt

1. In a large nonstick pot over medium-high heat, sauté the onions and garlic in ¼ cup of vegetable stock until softened.

2. Add the remaining 3¾ cups of stock, white mushrooms, portobello mushrooms, barley, carrot, celery, bouillon, soy sauce, pepper, and salt. Stir well, cover the pot, reduce the heat to medium low, and simmer for 40 minutes, or until the barley is plump and soft.

3. Store in the refrigerator for 5 to 7 days or in the freezer for 2 months.

Per serving: Calories: 143; Total fat: 1g; Carbohydrates: 30g; Fiber: 7g; Protein: 5g; Calcium: 5%; Vitamin D: 7%; Vitamin B$_{12}$: <1%; Iron: 9%; Zinc: 6%

Nutrition Tip: Choose pot barley (easily found in most grocery stores) over pearl barley, as it's less processed and retains the nutritious bran.

Maple-Garlic Air-Fried Tofu

Prep time: 5 minutes, plus
 10 minutes to marinate
Cook time: 20 minutes

SERVES 2

STRENGTH BUILDER | GLUTEN-FREE OPTION

NUT-FREE

Tofu is highly versatile and a great staple in the vegan kitchen. It comes in several forms—silken, soft, firm, and pressed (extra firm)—and it's packed with protein, calcium, iron, manganese, and selenium. This recipe uses firm tofu to create a sweet and spicy protein-rich dish.

2 tablespoons
 low-sodium soy sauce
 (or tamari, which is a
 gluten-free option)
¼ cup maple syrup

6 garlic cloves, minced
1 tablespoon apple
 cider vinegar
⅓ teaspoon
 ground ginger

⅛ teaspoon freshly
 ground black pepper
1 (350-gram) block firm
 tofu, cubed

1. In a medium bowl, combine the soy sauce, maple syrup, garlic, vinegar, ginger, and pepper and stir to mix well. Add the tofu and marinate for at least 10 minutes. The longer the tofu marinates, the more flavor it will absorb.

2. Put the tofu in the air fryer and cook for 18 to 20 minutes, or until the edges are crispy.

3. Enjoy immediately or store in the refrigerator for 5 to 7 days.

4. This goes well on a bed of brown rice or quinoa, with a side of steamed vegetables. Drizzle any excess marinade over the top.

Per serving: Calories: 314; Total fat: 10g; Carbohydrates: 38g; Fiber: 3g; Protein: 23g; Calcium: 18%; Vitamin D: 0%; Vitamin B$_{12}$: 0%; Iron: 23%; Zinc: 12%

Substitution Tip: If you don't have an air fryer, you can bake the tofu in the oven on a baking sheet lined with parchment paper or a silicone liner at 350°F for 20 to 25 minutes, or until the edges start to harden. The results won't be exactly the same, but the dish will still work well.

Lebanese-Inspired Yellow Beans and Rice

Prep time: 5 minutes
Cook time: 35 minutes
SERVES 4

RECOVERY **GLUTEN-FREE** **NUT-FREE**

This is a veganized version of a traditional Lebanese recipe my mom used to make. Ground cinnamon gives the dish its distinctive flavor and aroma. Cinnamon isn't just for sweets!

1 medium
  onion, chopped
3 garlic cloves, chopped
¾ cup water, divided
4 cups cooked
  brown rice
1 (28-ounce) can
  diced tomatoes

3 cups trimmed
  and halved fresh
  yellow beans
1 (19-ounce) can kidney
  beans, drained, rinsed,
  and roughly mashed
1½ teaspoons
  ground cinnamon

¼ teaspoon freshly
  ground black pepper
⅛ teaspoon pink
  Himalayan salt

1. In a large nonstick pan over medium-high heat, sauté the onion and garlic in ¼ cup of water for 10 minutes, or until softened.

2. Add the remaining ½ cup of water, the rice, tomatoes, yellow beans, kidney beans, cinnamon, pepper, and salt. Reduce the heat to medium low, stir, cover, and cook, stirring frequently, for 25 minutes, or until the yellow beans are soft. Serve immediately.

Per serving: Calories: 413; Total fat: 3g; Carbohydrates: 82g; Fiber: 17g; Protein: 15g; Calcium: 12%; Vitamin D: 0%; Vitamin B$_{12}$: 0%; Iron: 18%; Zinc: 7%

Substitution Tip: If fresh yellow beans are not available, you can use canned instead. The cooking time will be shorter because they are already soft.

Storage Tip: This stores well in the refrigerator for up to 5 days and makes a great meal prep option.

Orange-Ginger Stir-Fry

Prep time: 5 minutes
Cook time: 15 minutes
SERVES 2

ENERGY BOOST **GLUTEN-FREE** **NUT-FREE**

The fusion of fresh orange and ginger creates a delicious sauce to enjoy over vegetables and a bed of rice. Switch it up by using different vegetables, such as snap peas. Look for vegetables that are in season or on sale to keep this dish budget-friendly.

2 cups chopped broccoli

1 cup chopped mushrooms

1 red bell pepper, chopped

¼ cup water

1 cup orange juice

2 tablespoons low-sodium soy sauce (or tamari, which is a gluten-free option)

1½ tablespoons brown sugar

¼ tablespoon red pepper flakes

2-inch fresh ginger root, minced

2 teaspoons cornstarch

2 cups cooked brown rice

Chopped scallion, for garnish (optional)

1. In a large nonstick pan over medium-high heat, sauté the broccoli, mushrooms, and bell pepper in the water for 5 minutes.

2. In a medium saucepan over medium-high heat, combine the orange juice, soy sauce, brown sugar, red pepper flakes, ginger, and cornstarch. Bring to a boil, then reduce to a simmer and stir for 3 to 5 minutes, or until the sauce thickens.

3. Pour half the thickened sauce over the vegetables in the pan and stir for 5 minutes to incorporate the flavors.

4. Put the vegetables on top of the cooked rice and drizzle the remaining sauce over the top. Garnish with the scallion (if using).

Per serving: Calories: 371; Total fat: 3g; Carbohydrates: 81g; Fiber: 8g; Protein: 11g; Calcium: 7%; Vitamin D: 7%; Vitamin B_{12}: <1%; Iron: 11%; Zinc: 4%

Recipe Tip: Looking to boost the protein? Try adding cubed tofu, tempeh, or chickpeas. Or replace the brown rice with quinoa.

Stuffed Peppers

Prep time: 10 minutes

Cook time: 55 minutes

SERVES 4

Stuffed peppers are great for meal prep, so add them to your rotation for the week and store them in reusable containers in the refrigerator for up to 5 days.

4 red bell peppers

¼ cup TVP (textured vegetable protein)

¼ cup boiling water

1 small yellow onion, chopped

2 garlic cloves, minced

¼ cup vegetable broth

3½ cups tomato sauce, divided

1 (19-ounce) can red kidney beans, drained and rinsed

1 cup cooked brown rice

1 teaspoon dried oregano

½ teaspoon dried parsley

⅛ teaspoon freshly ground black pepper

⅛ teaspoon Himalayan pink salt

1. Preheat the oven to 350°F.

2. Remove the tops, seeds, and insides of the bell peppers.

3. In a small bowl, mix the TVP with the boiling water. Set aside.

4. In a medium nonstick pan over medium-high heat, sauté the onion and garlic in the broth for 5 minutes, or until soft. Stir in ½ cup of tomato sauce, the kidney beans, rice, oregano, parsley, pepper, and salt and cook for another 5 minutes. Stir in the TVP.

5. Fill the bell peppers with the mixture. Place the stuffed peppers in a glass pan. Top with the remaining 3 cups of tomato sauce. Cover with aluminum foil and cook for 45 minutes, or until the peppers have softened.

Per serving: Calories: 296; Total fat: 2g; Carbohydrates: 59g; Fiber: 16g; Protein: 15g; Calcium: 9%; Vitamin D: 0%; Vitamin B_{12}: 0%; Iron: 27%; Zinc: 9%

Nutrition Tip: TVP, short for textured vegetable protein, is a meat substitute made of defatted soybean flour. It is low in fat, high in protein, and easy to prepare, and it has a similar texture to meat crumbles. It takes on any flavors it's cooked with, so it's very versatile.

Veggie Fajitas

Prep time: 5 minutes

Cook time: 10 minutes

SERVES 4

ENERGY BOOST   NUT-FREE

These Veggie Fajitas are packed with flavor from the spices, vegetables, and black beans. Wrap it all up in a whole wheat tortilla, and you've got a plant-powered meal in just minutes.

1 tablespoon chili powder

½ tablespoon garlic powder

1 teaspoon onion powder

½ teaspoon ground cumin

½ teaspoon paprika

½ teaspoon cayenne pepper

1 red onion, sliced

½ red bell pepper, sliced

½ green bell pepper, sliced

1 garlic clove, minced

¼ cup vegetable broth

2 cups cooked black beans

1 cup sliced mushrooms

8 (8-inch) whole wheat tortillas

1. In a small bowl, mix the chili powder, garlic powder, onion powder, cumin, paprika, and cayenne pepper.

2. In a medium nonstick pan over medium-high heat, sauté the onion, red and green bell peppers, and garlic in the broth for 5 minutes, covered, stirring occasionally. Add the seasoning mix, black beans, and mushrooms. Stir and cook for another 5 minutes.

3. Divide the veggies equally among the tortillas and enjoy immediately or store the veggies in the refrigerator for up to 5 days.

Per serving (2 fajitas): Calories: 827; Total fat: 14g; Carbohydrates: 145g; Fiber: 32g; Protein: 35g; Calcium: 41%; Vitamin D: 7%; Vitamin B$_{12}$: <1%; Iron: 53%; Zinc: 17%

Recipe Tip: Optional toppings include avocado, salsa, shredded lettuce, vegan sour cream, vegan cheese, jalapeño, fresh lime, and fresh cilantro.

Teriyaki Tofu and Veggies

Prep time: 10 minutes
Cook time: 20 minutes
SERVES 2

RECOVERY **GLUTEN-FREE OPTION**

A healthier alternative to takeout, this teriyaki meal hits the spot with a tasty sauce and fresh vegetables. Some traditional recipes call for medium or soft tofu, but I opt for firm because I prefer the texture and flavor. Use your favorite type of tofu, or experiment with different ones to see which one you like best.

½ cup low-sodium soy sauce (or tamari, which is a gluten-free option)

¾ cup water, divided, plus 1 tablespoon

1-inch fresh ginger root, minced

1 garlic clove, minced

1 tablespoon apple cider vinegar

1 tablespoon coconut sugar

½ tablespoon garlic powder

1 tablespoon cornstarch

½ (350-gram) block firm tofu, cubed

2 cups chopped broccoli

½ cup grated carrots

1 green bell pepper, chopped

1 cup snap peas

2 cups cooked brown rice

2 scallions, chopped, for garnish

Toasted sesame seeds, for garnish (optional)

1. In a small saucepan over medium-low heat, combine the soy sauce, ½ cup of water, ginger, garlic, vinegar, coconut sugar, and garlic powder. Stir continuously, until the teriyaki sauce begins to thicken. Set aside.

2. In a small bowl, mix the cornstarch and 1 tablespoon of water into a slurry, and add it to the saucepan. Continue to stir to thicken the mixture.

3. In a medium nonstick pan over medium-low heat, sauté the tofu, broccoli, carrots, bell pepper, and snap peas in the remaining ¼ cup of water. Cover and cook, stirring frequently and adding small amounts of water if needed, until the vegetables are soft.

4. Add the prepared teriyaki sauce, stirring to mix it thoroughly with the vegetables and tofu.

5. Serve the vegetables and tofu over the rice, garnished with the scallions and sesame seeds (if using).

Per serving: Calories: 479; Total fat: 7g; Carbohydrates: 81g; Fiber: 11g; Protein: 25g; Calcium: 16%; Vitamin D: 0%; Vitamin B_{12}: 0%; Iron: 21%; Zinc: 5%

Nutrition Tip: Did you know soy does not contain estrogen? The hormone is present only in meat and dairy. Soy contains phytoestrogen, which is found in plants and is not the same as its animal-based counterpart.

Turmeric Italian Tofu and Rice

Prep time: 5 minutes
Cook time: 30 Minutes

SERVES 2

PRE-GAME GLUTEN-FREE NUT-FREE

Take this meal with you for lunch or enjoy it after your training session to make sure you get quality protein and carbs. Looking for iron and even more protein? Swap out the brown rice for quinoa.

For the rice

2 cups water
1 cup uncooked brown rice
1 cup vegetable broth
1 garlic clove, minced
1 teaspoon dried oregano
⅛ teaspoon turmeric
⅛ teaspoon pink Himalayan salt
⅛ teaspoon freshly ground black pepper

For the tofu and vegetables

1 (350-gram) block firm tofu, chopped
½ cup vegetable broth
½ cup chopped zucchini
½ cup diced red onion
½ cup chopped red bell pepper
1 medium fresh tomato, chopped
1 garlic clove, minced
½ teaspoon dried oregano
⅛ teaspoon turmeric
⅛ teaspoon freshly ground black pepper

To make the rice

1. In a large pot over high heat, combine the water, the rice, broth, garlic, oregano, turmeric, salt, and pepper. Bring to a boil. Reduce the heat to low and simmer, covered, for 20 to 25 minutes, or until the rice is soft. Note: Some brown rice may require an additional ½ cup of water.

To make the tofu and vegetables

2. In a medium nonstick skillet over medium heat, combine all the ingredients and cook for 10 minutes, stirring frequently, until soft.

3. Serve on top of the brown rice.

Per serving: Calories: 381; Total fat: 9g; Carbohydrates: 61g; Fiber: 7g; Protein: 21g; Calcium: 13%; Vitamin D: 0%; Vitamin B$_{12}$: 0%; Iron: 23%; Zinc: 2%

Shepherd's Pie

Prep time: 15 minutes

Cook time: 35 minutes

SERVES 4

RECOVERY GLUTEN-FREE NUT-FREE

You can't go wrong with this hearty lentil-and-potato meal packed with vegetables in a savory gravy sauce. And no one will miss the meat!

1 medium yellow onion, diced

2 garlic cloves, minced

1¼ cups vegetable broth, divided

3 cups cooked or canned lentils (drained and rinsed, if canned)

½ cup frozen peas

½ cup frozen carrots

½ cup frozen green beans

½ cup frozen corn

⅛ teaspoon freshly ground black pepper, plus ½ teaspoon

1½ teaspoons dried rosemary

1½ teaspoons vegan Worcestershire sauce (check label for gluten-free)

1 teaspoon tomato paste

5 to 6 medium yellow potatoes

½ cup unsweetened plant-based milk

2 tablespoons whole wheat flour

Pink Himalayan salt (optional)

Smoked paprika (optional)

1. Preheat the oven to 350°F.

2. In a large nonstick pan over medium-high heat, sauté the onion and garlic in ½ cup vegetable broth for 5 minutes, or until soft. Stir in the lentils, peas, carrots, green beans, corn, whole wheat flour, and the remaining ¾ cup of broth. Add ⅛ teaspoon of pepper, the rosemary, Worcestershire sauce, and tomato paste. Cover, reduce the heat to medium low, and cook, stirring occasionally, for 10 minutes.

3. While the vegetables are cooking, in a large pot over high heat, boil the potatoes for 15 minutes, until soft. Drain and mash with the milk and remaining ½ teaspoon of pepper. Add salt to taste (if using).

(continued)

Shepherd's Pie (continued)

4. In a 9-by-13-inch casserole dish, evenly spread the vegetable mixture. Spread the mashed potatoes on top. Sprinkle with paprika (if using).

5. Cook for 20 minutes, or until the mashed potatoes on top are lightly browned.

Per serving: Calories: 382; Total fat: 1g; Carbohydrates: 77g; Fiber: 18g; Protein: 20g; Calcium: 14%; Vitamin D: 3%; Vitamin B$_{12}$: 0%; Iron: 40%; Zinc: 18%

Prep Tip: Include this well-balanced recipe in your meal prep by dividing it into equal parts and storing them in reusable containers in the refrigerator for 5 to 7 days.

Substitution Tip: To switch it up, try swapping out these mashed potatoes for Garlic Cauliflower Mashed Potatoes (page 118).

Spaghetti & Meat-Free Meatballs

Prep time: 10 minutes

Cook time: 25 minutes

SERVES 4

STRENGTH BUILDER | **GLUTEN-FREE**

The seasonings in this recipe bring back the familiar flavors of this classic Italian food, with the added benefit of fiber that you don't get with the meat-based version.

½ cup TVP (textured vegetable protein)

½ cup boiling water

2 cups cooked black beans

1 cup rolled oats (check label for gluten-free), blended to a flour consistency

1 garlic clove, minced

½ small yellow onion, diced

½ cup cremini mushrooms

3 tablespoons aquafaba (the liquid from a can of chickpeas)

1 teaspoon Italian seasoning

½ teaspoon ground flaxseed

½ teaspoon dried oregano

½ teaspoon dried basil

Fresh parsley, for garnish (optional)

Parmesan Cheese (page 183), for topping

1. Preheat the oven to 350°F. Line a baking sheet with parchment paper or a silicone liner.

2. In a small bowl, mix the TVP with the boiling water and let it sit for 5 minutes.

3. In a food processor, combine the TVP, beans, oats, garlic, onion, mushrooms, aquafaba, Italian seasoning, flaxseed, oregano, and basil and pulse until the ingredients are well mixed but not smooth. Don't overblend. (Here's a trick to avoid overblending: after a few pulses, finish mixing with a wooden spoon.)

4. Using your hands, form the mixture into 2-inch balls and place them on the prepared baking sheet. Cook for 20 to 25 minutes, or until lightly browned.

5. Serve with your favorite chickpea-based spaghetti and sauce, topped with parsley and Parmesan cheese (if using).

Per serving (4 meat-free balls): Calories: 316; Total fat: 3g; Carbohydrates: 52g; Fiber: 16g; Protein: 22g; Calcium: 5%; Vitamin D: 2%; Vitamin B$_{12}$: <1%; Iron: 23%; Zinc: 10%

Meat-Free Loaf

Prep time: 10 minutes

Cook time: 50 minutes

SERVES 6

STRENGTH BUILDER   GLUTEN-FREE   NUT-FREE

This veganized classic has all the flavors you remember but without the meat. It's a healthy meat alternative; no junk here, just wholesome ingredients packed with nutrients and plant-based protein.

¾ cup rolled oats (check label for gluten-free)

4 cups cooked lentils, divided

2 cups chopped mushrooms

2 celery stalks, finely chopped

1 medium onion, diced

2 garlic cloves, minced

¼ cup plus 2 tablespoons water

½ cup chickpea flour

2 tablespoons dried basil

1 teaspoon onion powder

1 teaspoon garlic powder

¼ teaspoon pink Himalayan salt

¼ cup organic ketchup

½ tablespoon balsamic vinegar

½ tablespoon brown sugar

1. Preheat the oven to 350°F. Line a loaf pan with parchment paper or a silicone liner.

2. Put the oats in a food processor and pulse a few times to roughly break them down. Transfer to a large bowl.

3. Put 2 cups of lentils in the food processor and pulse a few times. Transfer to the bowl with the oats.

4. In a medium nonstick pan over medium-high heat, sauté the mushrooms, celery, onion, and garlic in ¼ cup of water until the onion is tender. Transfer to the bowl.

5. Add the flour, remaining 2 cups of lentils, basil, onion powder, garlic powder, and salt to the bowl and mix well to combine all the ingredients.

6. Transfer the mixture to the prepared pan and form it into a loaf shape.

7. In a small bowl, combine 2 tablespoons of water, the ketchup, vinegar, and brown sugar. Spread the sauce on top of the loaf.

8. Cook for 45 minutes, or until the edges of the loaf are slightly crispy. Serve immediately or store in the refrigerator for up to 5 days.

Per serving: Calories: 386; Total fat: 3g; Carbohydrates: 70g; Fiber: 21g; Protein: 24g; Calcium: 11%; Vitamin D: 7%; Vitamin B$_{12}$: <1%; Iron: 51%; Zinc: 20%

Recipe Tip: To make a full plate, serve this loaf with Garlic Cauliflower Mashed Potatoes (page 118) and Creamy Green Beans (page 111).

Ricotta Red Sauce Pasta

Prep time: 5 minutes, plus
   1 hour to soak the cashews
Cook time: 25 minutes

SERVES 4

If you love pasta, ricotta, and tomato sauce, this dish hits the mark, all without dairy. This is a great choice when you're looking for a deeply satisfying meal.

1 (350-gram) block
   firm tofu
1 cup cashews, soaked
   for 1 hour in hot water
1 cup fresh spinach
1 cup chopped
   mushrooms
4 garlic cloves
1½ tablespoons
   B_{12}-fortified
   nutritional yeast

1 tablespoon freshly
   squeezed lemon juice
1 teaspoon
   dried oregano
½ teaspoon dried basil
¼ teaspoon pink
   Himalayan salt
⅛ teaspoon freshly
   ground black pepper

10 ounces
   chickpea-based pasta
1½ cups vegan red
   pasta sauce
Parmesan Cheese
   (page 183), for
   topping (optional)

1. In a food processor, blend the tofu, cashews, spinach, mushrooms, garlic, nutritional yeast, lemon juice, oregano, basil, salt, and pepper until smooth.

2. In a large pot of boiling water, cook the pasta according to the package instructions. Drain.

3. In a large nonstick pan over medium-low heat, combine the cashew ricotta with the pasta sauce and cook for 5 minutes. Add the pasta and stir. Sprinkle with Parmesan cheese (if using). Serve immediately.

Per serving: Calories: 610; Total fat: 28g; Carbohydrates: 66g; Fiber: 16g; Protein: 36g; Calcium: 16%; Vitamin D: 3%; Vitamin B_{12}: 19%; Iron: 67%; Zinc: 17%

Storage Tip: This stores well in an airtight container in the refrigerator for 3 to 5 days.

Classic Lasagna

Prep time: 20 minutes, plus 1 hour
   to soak the cashews
Cook time: 25 minutes

SERVES 4

When I first went vegan in 2011, the Italian side of me knew I had to veganize my lasagna. Not only is this one of my all-time favorite meals, but I also get requests to bring this vegan dish to family gatherings and holiday dinners. One of the best ways to teach people about the vegan lifestyle is to feed them delicious food!

For the filling

1½ cups cashews,
   soaked in hot water for
   at least 1 hour
1⅓ cups water
1 tablespoon freshly
   squeezed lemon juice
1 tablespoon
   white vinegar

2 tablespoons
   tapioca flour
1 teaspoon pink
   Himalayan salt

For the lasagna

1 (375-gram) box
   lasagna noodles
1 small onion, diced
2 garlic cloves, chopped

2¾ cups water, divided
1½ cups TVP (textured
   vegetable protein)
3 to 4 cups vegan red
   pasta sauce
2 cups sliced
   fresh mushrooms
2 cups fresh spinach

To make the filling

1. In the food processor, combine all the ingredients and blend until liquid and completely smooth, with no remaining lumps.

2. In a nonstick pot over medium heat, cook the mixture for 10 to 15 minutes, continuously stirring. The mixture will start to thicken and become stretchy. Once thickened, remove from the heat and pour into a glass container.

(continued)

Classic Lasagna (continued)

To make the lasagna

3. Preheat the oven to 350°F.

4. In a large pot over high heat, cook the lasagna noodles to al dente according to the package instructions.

5. In a medium nonstick pan over medium heat, sauté the onion and garlic in ¼ cup of water for 5 minutes, or until soft. Add the TVP and the remaining 2½ cups of water and continue to cook until the TVP is hydrated and soft. Add the pasta sauce and stir together.

6. In a 9-by-13-inch glass casserole dish, spread a small layer of sauce. Top with a layer of noodles. Add a layer of the TVP sauce and a layer of mushrooms and spinach. Repeat the layers with the remaining ingredients.

7. Cover with aluminum foil and cook for 20 minutes.

8. Serve immediately or store in the refrigerator in a reusable container for up to 5 days.

Per serving: Calories: 910; Total fat: 30g; Carbohydrates: 116g; Fiber: 16g; Protein: 41g; Calcium: 5%; Vitamin D: 7%; Vitamin B$_{12}$: <1%; Iron: 46%; Zinc: 21%

Recipe Tip: This lasagna goes deliciously well with Caesar Salad (page 89).

Ultimate Cheesy Mac

Prep time: 15 minutes
Cook time: 15 minutes

SERVES 2

ENERGY BOOST   **GLUTEN-FREE**   **NUT-FREE**

It's truly amazing what we can create with plants. A cheese made with potatoes and carrots that's nut-free, too? Yes! And it's absolutely delicious. It's sure to satisfy your mac and cheese cravings, all with easy-to-find ingredients. This will store well in the refrigerator for 3 days, although there's rarely enough left to store.

2 cups peeled chopped potatoes

1 cup peeled chopped carrots

½ cup unsweetened plant-based milk

½ cup B$_{12}$-fortified nutritional yeast

2 teaspoons pink Himalayan salt

¼ teaspoon onion powder

¼ teaspoon garlic powder

1 tablespoon freshly squeezed lemon juice

⅛ teaspoon ground turmeric

6 ounces chickpea-based pasta, or pasta of choice

1. In a medium pot over medium-high heat, boil the potatoes and carrots for 10 minutes. Make sure not to overcook them, as that will affect the texture of the sauce.

2. Transfer the vegetables to a food processor and add the milk, nutritional yeast, salt, onion powder, garlic powder, lemon juice, and turmeric and blend until smooth.

3. In a medium pot over high heat, cook the pasta according to the package instructions, then drain.

4. Pour the cheesy sauce over the pasta and enjoy immediately.

Per serving: Calories: 547; Total fat: 8g; Carbohydrates: 99g; Fiber: 24g; Protein: 38g; Calcium: 23%; Vitamin D: 8%; Vitamin B$_{12}$: 213%; Iron: 60%; Zinc: 38%

Substitution Tip: Make this into a queso dip. Add 1 to 2 tablespoons of chopped jalapeño peppers and ¼ cup salsa when blending the cheese in the food processor.

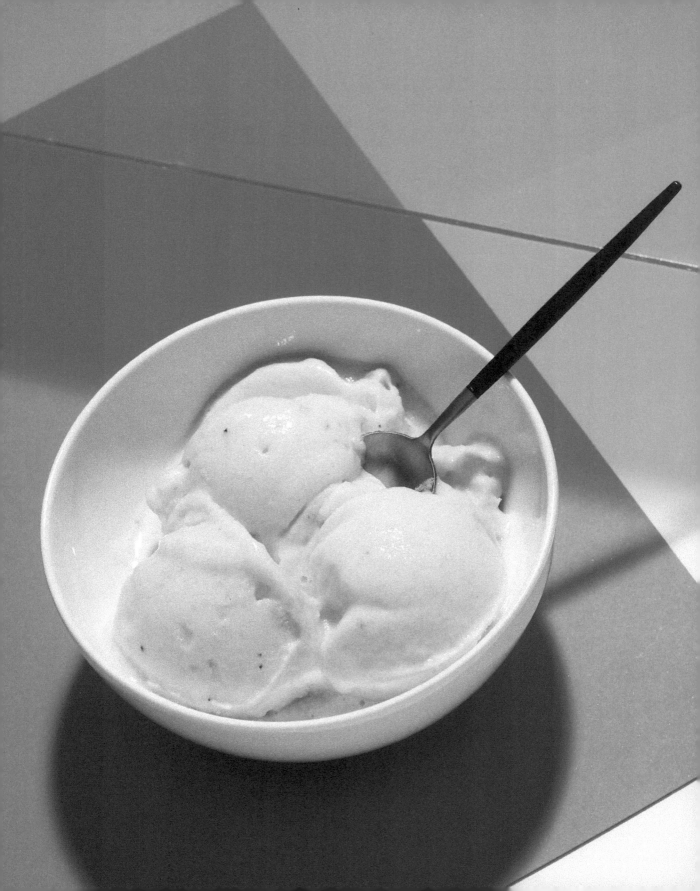

CHAPTER 8

Desserts

Orange Nice Cream, 169

Banana Chocolate Chip Cookies

Prep time: 5 minutes

Cook time: 10 minutes

MAKES 9 COOKIES

GRAB AND GO　GLUTEN-FREE

This quick, no-fuss cookie recipe uses very few ingredients. It's budget-friendly, tasty, and the perfect snack or dessert when you are craving something sweet but don't want junk food.

2 bananas

1 cup rolled oats (check label for gluten-free)

1 teaspoon ground flaxseed

1 teaspoon vanilla extract

¼ cup vegan mini chocolate chips

¼ cup chopped walnuts

1. Preheat the oven to 350°F. Line a baking sheet with parchment paper or a silicone liner.

2. In a food processor, combine the bananas, oats, flaxseed, and vanilla and blend until very well combined. Use a wooden spoon to stir in the chocolate chips and walnuts.

3. Scoop the batter into 9 cookies, spacing them out on the prepared baking sheet. Bake for 8 to 12 minutes, or until the bottoms are light brown. Enjoy right after they cool or store in a reusable container at room temperature.

Per serving (1 cookie): Calories: 112; Total fat: 5g; Carbohydrates: 17g; Fiber: 2g; Protein: 2g; Calcium: 1%; Vitamin D: 0%; Vitamin B$_{12}$: 0%; Iron: 3%; Zinc: 1%

Substitution Tip: Try swapping out the walnuts for your favorite nuts, seeds, or dried fruit.

Banana-Walnut Bread

Prep time: 5 minutes

Cook time: 50 minutes

SERVES 6

This banana bread is soft on the inside with a subtly sweet taste and a little crunch from the chopped walnuts. Slice it and add it to your snack options for the week. Or enjoy a piece when you're on the go and need a quick bite between meals.

2 cups whole wheat flour

¾ teaspoon baking soda

3 very ripe bananas, mashed

½ cup maple syrup

¼ cup unsweetened applesauce

6 tablespoons aquafaba (the liquid from a can of chickpeas)

1 teaspoon vanilla extract

1 teaspoon pink Himalayan salt

¾ cup chopped walnuts

1. Preheat the oven to 350°F. Line a loaf pan with parchment paper or a silicone liner.

2. In a mixing bowl, sift together the flour and baking soda.

3. In a separate bowl, combine the mashed bananas, maple syrup, applesauce, aquafaba, vanilla, and salt. Mix well. Stir in the flour mixture and mix well. Gently stir in the walnuts.

4. Pour the mixture into the prepared pan. Bake for 40 to 50 minutes, until brown on the top and edges. Enjoy right after it cools or store in a reusable container at room temperature for up to 5 days.

Per serving: Calories: 541; Total fat: 17g; Carbohydrates: 96g; Fiber: 11g; Protein: 12g; Calcium: 5%; Vitamin D: 0%; Vitamin B_{12}: 0%; Iron: 8%; Zinc: 17%

Substitution Tip: You can swap out the chopped walnuts for sunflower seeds, pumpkin seeds, or vegan dark chocolate chips.

Black Bean & Walnut Brownie Bites

Prep time: 10 minutes
Cook time: 40 minutes
MAKES 12 BITES

GRAB AND GO   GLUTEN-FREE OPTION

This recipe just might surprise you. It's perfect when you're craving chocolate and want a healthier choice.

1 (19-ounce) can black beans, drained and rinsed

2½ tablespoons maple syrup

2 tablespoons coconut sugar

2 teaspoons vanilla extract

2 tablespoons unsweetened applesauce

2 tablespoons whole wheat flour (or gluten-free flour)

1 tablespoon unsweetened plant-based milk

2 teaspoons cocoa powder

½ teaspoon baking powder

½ teaspoon baking soda

½ cup mini vegan dark chocolate chips

¼ cup chopped walnuts

1. Preheat the oven to 350°F. Insert silicone muffin cups into a muffin pan.

2. In a food processor, combine the black beans, maple syrup, coconut sugar, vanilla, applesauce, flour, milk, cocoa powder, baking powder, and baking soda. Blend until mixed well and mostly smooth.

3. Pour the mixture into a bowl and stir in the chocolate chips and walnuts.

4. Fill each muffin cup about half full of batter. Bake for 40 minutes, or until a toothpick inserted into the center of a brownie bite comes out clean. Enjoy as soon as they cool or store in a reusable container in the refrigerator for up to 5 days.

Per serving (1 bite): Calories: 128; Total fat: 5g; Carbohydrates: 20g; Fiber: 4g; Protein: 3g; Calcium: 3%; Vitamin D: <1%; Vitamin B$_{12}$: <1%; Iron: 4%; Zinc: 4%

Chewy Cashew Bars

Prep time: 5 minutes

Cook time: 15 minutes

MAKES 10 BARS

If you're looking for a healthy and satisfying snack that's great any time, before or after training, this is the one. Add these nutrient-packed bars to your meal prep rotation for the week ahead so you'll be prepared when hunger strikes between meals.

10 Medjool dates, pitted

1 cup cashews

1 cup cooked chickpeas (drained and rinsed, if canned)

2 tablespoons sunflower seeds

2 tablespoons pumpkin seeds

2 teaspoons vanilla extract

8 ounces vegan dark mini chocolate chips

1. Line a baking sheet with parchment paper or a silicone liner.

2. In a food processor, combine the dates, cashews, chickpeas, sunflower seeds, pumpkin seeds, and vanilla. Blend, but leave the mixture a little chunky.

3. Shape the mixture into bars and place them on the prepared baking sheet. Bake for 15 minutes, or until the edges become lightly browned. Remove from the oven and let cool for 10 minutes.

4. In a small saucepan over low heat, stir the chocolate chips until melted. Coat the top of the bars with the melted chocolate and let cool to room temperature.

Per serving (1 bar): Calories: 299; Total fat: 15g; Carbohydrates: 42g; Fiber: 5g; Protein: 5g; Calcium: 3%; Vitamin D: 0%; Vitamin B_{12}: 0%; Iron: 9%; Zinc: 8%

Storage Tip: Store in a reusable container in the refrigerator for up to 7 days.

Chocolate-Avocado Pudding

Prep time: 5 minutes

SERVES 2

Chocolate pudding made with avocados? Seems like an unlikely combination, but they work really well together. The healthy essential fats from the avocado make this pudding smooth and rich without dominating the flavor. This pudding is delicious on its own, or you can enjoy it with some mixed nuts or topped with Maple Crunch Granola (page 104).

2 ripe avocados, pitted and peeled

¼ cup unsweetened plant-based milk

⅓ cup coconut sugar

⅓ cup cocoa powder

1 teaspoon vanilla extract

▶ In a food processor, combine all the ingredients and blend until you achieve a smooth pudding consistency. Serve immediately.

Per serving: Calories: 457; Total fat: 29g; Carbohydrates: 56g; Fiber: 17g; Protein: 6g; Calcium: 10%; Vitamin D: 3%; Vitamin B$_{12}$: 0%; Iron: 17%; Zinc: 14%

Recipe Tip: This pudding should be enjoyed immediately, or at least on the same day you make it.

Cranberry-Almond Muffins

Prep time: 10 minutes, plus 1 hour to soak the cranberries

Cook time: 20 minutes

MAKES 12 MUFFINS

This tasty snack delivers a subtle hint of maple sweetness in a fluffy muffin with cranberry and almond pieces throughout.

2 cups whole wheat flour (or gluten-free flour)

1 teaspoon baking soda

1 teaspoon baking powder

½ teaspoon pink Himalayan salt

1 cup unsweetened plant-based milk

¾ cup dried cranberries, soaked in water for 1 hour to soften

½ cup maple syrup

¼ cup chopped almonds

⅓ cup unsweetened applesauce

4 tablespoons freshly squeezed lemon juice

3 tablespoons aquafaba (the liquid from a can of chickpeas)

½ teaspoon vanilla extract

1. Preheat the oven to 375°F. Insert silicone muffin cups into a muffin pan.

2. In a bowl, combine the flour, baking soda, baking powder, and salt and mix well.

3. In a separate bowl, combine the milk, cranberries, maple syrup, almonds, applesauce, lemon juice, aquafaba, and vanilla and mix well.

4. Combine the wet and dry ingredients and mix well.

5. Fill each muffin cup a little more than half full with batter. Bake for 20 minutes, or until lightly browned and a toothpick inserted into the center of a muffin comes out clean. Enjoy as soon as they cool or store in a reusable container at room temperature.

Per serving (1 muffin): Calories: 143; Total fat: 2g; Carbohydrates: 31g; Fiber: 3g; Protein: 3g; Calcium: 9%; Vitamin D: 2%; Vitamin B$_{12}$: 0%; Iron: 6%; Zinc: 4%

Recipe Tip: Remove the muffins from the silicone inserts as soon as they are cool enough to handle to prevent condensation from building up in the inserts and giving the muffins soggy bottoms.

No-Bake Chocolate Chip Bites

Prep time: 10 minutes

MAKES 10 BITES

GRAB AND GO | **GLUTEN-FREE OPTION**

What's better than no-bake, no-fuss little chocolate chip bites? Make a quick batch and have these snacks on deck when you're rushing out the door or just on the prowl for a healthy snack.

¼ cup rolled oats (check label for gluten-free)

½ cup cashews

3 tablespoons whole wheat flour (or gluten-free flour)

½ teaspoon ground flaxseed

¼ teaspoon Himalayan pink salt

2 tablespoons maple syrup

1 teaspoon vanilla extract

2 tablespoons vegan dark chocolate chips

1. In a food processor, combine the oats, cashews, flour, flaxseed, and salt. When the dry ingredients are fully mixed, add the maple syrup and vanilla and continue to mix in the processor.

2. Add the chocolate chips and mix them in with a spoon. Using your hands, shape the mixture into 1-inch balls. Enjoy immediately or store in a reusable container in the refrigerator for up to 5 days.

Per serving (1 bite): Calories: 81; Total fat: 4g; Carbohydrates: 10g; Fiber: 1g; Protein: 2g; Calcium: 1%; Vitamin D: 0%; Vitamin B_{12}: 0%; Iron: 4%; Zinc: 4%

Substitution Tip: You can replace the chocolate chips with raisins, chopped dried apricots, or other dried fruits. Also, try adding coconut shreds to the mix to switch it up.

Orange Nice Cream

Prep time: 5 minutes

SERVES 1

ENERGY BOOST   GLUTEN-FREE   NUT-FREE

This easy-to-make and healthy soft-serve treat is a delicious and creamy alternative to ice cream. Try topping it with vegan dark chocolate chips, fresh fruit, or Maple Crunch Granola (page 104).

1 orange, peeled, separated into segments, and frozen

2 bananas, peeled, sliced, and frozen

½ teaspoon vanilla extract

¼ teaspoon hemp seeds

▶ In a food processor or blender, combine all the ingredients and blend until smooth and creamy. Enjoy immediately or store in a reusable container in the freezer for up to 1 month.

Per serving: Calories: 283; Total fat: 1g; Carbohydrates: 70g; Fiber: 9g; Protein: 4g; Calcium: 7%; Vitamin D: 0%; Vitamin B_{12}: 1%; Iron: 5%; Zinc: 4%

Substitution Tip: Try switching up the flavors by swapping out the oranges with pieces of frozen pineapple, strawberries, blueberries, or any combinations of your favorite fruits.

Pineapple-Coconut Macaroons

Prep time: 5 minutes

Cook time: 20 minutes

MAKES 10 MACAROONS

GRAB AND GO   **GLUTEN-FREE OPTION**

An irresistible combination of tropical flavors from a perfect blend of coconut, pineapple, and banana, these sweet treats with a chewy middle skip the eggs and dairy but not the flavor.

1⅓ cups unsweetened coconut shreds

½ cup chopped pineapple

½ cup coconut sugar

½ banana

3 tablespoons wheat flour (or gluten-free flour)

1. Preheat the oven to 350°F. Line a baking sheet with parchment paper or a silicone liner.

2. In a food processor, combine all the ingredients and process until almost smooth.

3. Use a tablespoon to make 10 heaping macaroons. Space them evenly on the prepared baking sheet.

4. Bake for 20 minutes, or until the tops and bottoms are light brown.

5. Let cool on a wire rack for 10 minutes before serving. Store in a reusable container in the refrigerator for up to 5 days.

Per serving (1 macaroon): Calories: 90; Total fat: 4g; Carbohydrates: 15g; Fiber: 1g; Protein: 1g; Calcium: <1%; Vitamin D: 0%; Vitamin B$_{12}$: 0%; Iron: 2%; Zinc: 1%

Substitution Tip: Try dipping the bottoms of the macaroons in melted vegan dark chocolate or drizzling melted chocolate on top.

Sweet and Salty Chocolate Bark

Prep time: 5 minutes
Cook time: 5 minutes

SERVES 6

GRAB AND GO   GLUTEN-FREE

This treat will satisfy your sweet tooth, your craving for a touch of salt, and your yen for some crunch. Try different combinations of nuts, seeds, and dried fruits to switch up the flavors. This is the perfect chocolate snack when you're on the go, at work, or at home.

¼ cup dried cranberries

3 tablespoons chopped pistachios

3 tablespoons chopped almonds

3 tablespoons pumpkin seeds

3 tablespoons sunflower seeds

1 (8-ounce) bag vegan dark chocolate chips

Pink Himalayan salt

1. Line an 8-inch square baking pan with parchment paper. Spread out the cranberries, pistachios, almonds, pumpkin seeds, and sunflower seeds on the baking pan.

2. In a small nonstick saucepan on low heat, gently heat the chocolate chips, stirring continuously, until they are melted and smooth.

3. Pour the melted chocolate evenly over the nuts, seeds, and dried fruit in the baking pan. Let cool to room temperature. Sprinkle with salt. Break the bark into pieces and remove from the baking pan.

Per serving: Calories: 275; Total fat: 18g; Carbohydrates: 30g; Fiber: 4g; Protein: 4g; Calcium: 2%; Vitamin D: 0%; Vitamin B$_{12}$: 0%; Iron: 4%; Zinc: 2%

Storage Tip: Store in a reusable container at room temperature for up to 14 days.

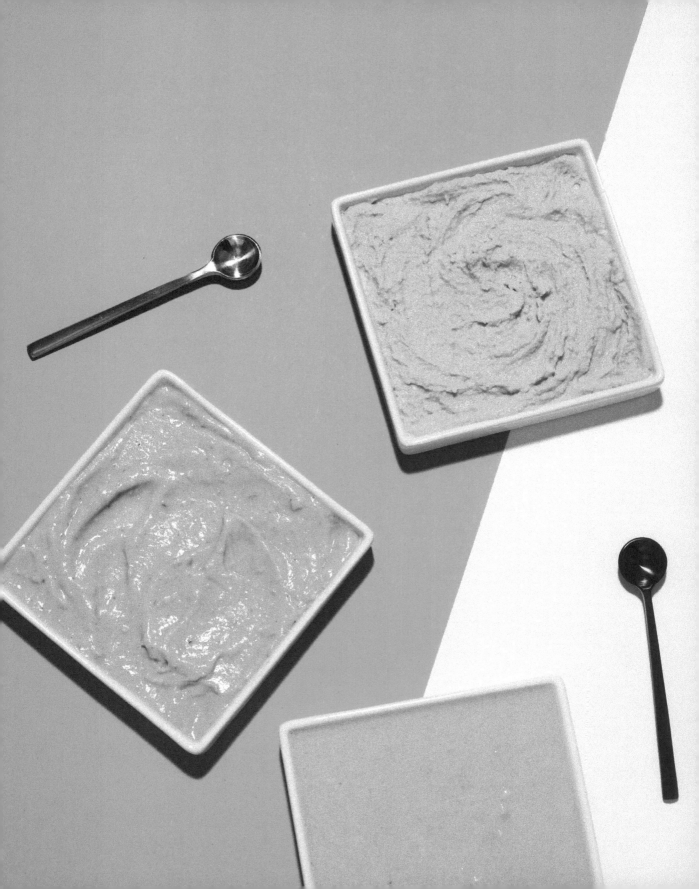

CHAPTER 9 Staples, Sauces, and Dressings

Turmeric Hummus (top), 184; Creamy Avocado Dressing (left), 177;
Lemon-Garlic Tahini (bottom), 181

Electrolyte Sports Drink

Prep time: 5 minutes

SERVES 1

RECOVERY   GLUTEN-FREE

I've been using this homemade, all-natural alternative to store-bought sports drinks for years. It's a delicious way to replenish your electrolytes and rehydrate. It's easy to make and much healthier than sugar-packed versions.

1 cup water

1 cup coconut water

1 cup orange juice

Juice of ½ lime

Juice of ½ lemon

¼ teaspoon pink Himalayan salt

▶ In a large Mason jar or sports bottle, combine all the ingredients and shake or stir to mix well. Enjoy immediately or store in the refrigerator for up to 10 days.

Per serving: Calories: 163; Total fat: 1g; Carbohydrates: 34g; Fiber: 1g; Protein: 2g; Calcium: 8%; Vitamin D: 0%; Vitamin B$_{12}$: 0%; Iron: 2%; Zinc: 1%

Nutrition Tip: It's critical that athletes replenish the electrolytes they lose through physical activity. Some of the symptoms you may experience if you don't replenish are muscle cramping, fatigue, dizziness, and headaches.

Prep Tip: Take this drink with you in a sealed Mason jar or sports bottle and consume during or right after training.

Pico de Gallo

Prep time: 5 minutes

SERVES 2

Pico de gallo is similar to salsa, but in my opinion, it's so much better! It's much chunkier than salsa, so each freshly chopped ingredient is distinctly visible and flavorful. Enjoy it with your nachos and tacos, or on top of a baked potato, for an incredible freshness that just makes whatever you're eating even more delicious.

3 large tomatoes, chopped

½ small red onion, diced

⅛ cup chopped fresh cilantro

3 garlic cloves, chopped

2 tablespoons chopped pickled jalapeño pepper

1 tablespoon lime juice

¼ teaspoon pink Himalayan salt (optional)

▶ In a medium bowl, combine all the ingredients and mix with a wooden spoon.

Per serving: Calories: 77; Total fat: 1g; Carbohydrates: 16g; Fiber: 4g; Protein: 3g; Calcium: 3%; Vitamin D: 0%; Vitamin B_{12}: 0%; Iron: 9%; Zinc: 3%

Storage Tip: Pico de gallo is best enjoyed fresh, but you can store it in the refrigerator for up to 3 days.

Sweet Ginger Sauce

Prep time: 5 minutes

Cook time: 5 minutes

MAKES ABOUT ⅔ CUP

This quick and easy-to-make dipping sauce is perfect with Air-Fried Spring Rolls (page 76) or countless other finger foods. It has a wonderful sweetness with a kick of fresh ginger.

3 tablespoons ketchup

2 tablespoons water

2 tablespoons
maple syrup

1 tablespoon
rice vinegar

2 teaspoons peeled
minced fresh
ginger root

2 teaspoons soy sauce
(or tamari, which is a
gluten-free option)

1 teaspoon cornstarch

▶ In a small saucepan over medium heat, combine all the ingredients and stir continuously for 5 minutes, or until slightly thickened. Enjoy warm or cold.

Per serving (⅓ cup): Calories: 92; Total fat: <1g; Carbohydrates: 23g; Fiber: <1g; Protein: <1g; Calcium: 2%; Vitamin D: 0%; Vitamin B$_{12}$: 0%; Iron: 2%; Zinc: 6%

Storage Tip: Store leftover sauce in a reusable container in the refrigerator for up to 14 days.

Creamy Avocado Dressing

Prep time: 5 minutes

MAKES 12 TABLESPOONS

This creamy and rich dressing is really versatile. It goes well with many different types of salads, sides, or even drizzled on top of Loaded Baked Sweet Potatoes (page 122). It's a delicious and refreshingly light alternative to oil-based dressings.

1 large avocado, pitted and peeled

½ cup water

2 tablespoons tahini

2 tablespoons freshly squeezed lemon juice

1 teaspoon dried basil

1 teaspoon white wine vinegar

1 garlic clove

¼ teaspoon pink Himalayan salt

¼ teaspoon freshly ground black pepper

▶ Combine all the ingredients in a food processor and blend until smooth.

Per serving (1 tablespoon): Calories: 43; Total fat: 4g; Carbohydrates: 2g; Fiber: 2g; Protein: 1g; Calcium: 2%; Vitamin D: 0%; Vitamin B$_{12}$: 0%; Iron: 2%; Zinc: 1%

Storage Tip: This dressing is best enjoyed immediately or on the same day you make it. But, if necessary, you can store it in a container in the refrigerator for up to 2 days.

Dijon Balsamic Vinaigrette

Prep time: 5 minutes

MAKES 12 TABLESPOONS

GLUTEN-FREE   NUT-FREE

With its tangy, tasty, robust flavor, you can whip up this no-fuss vinaigrette quickly. It's delicious on salad or as a marinade for vegetables or grilled tofu.

6 tablespoons water

4 tablespoons
  Dijon mustard

4 tablespoons
  balsamic vinegar

1 teaspoon maple syrup

½ teaspoon pink
  Himalayan salt

¼ teaspoon freshly
  ground black pepper

▶   In a bowl, whisk together all the ingredients.

Per serving (1 tablespoon): Calories: 18; Total fat: 1g; Carbohydrates: 1g; Fiber: 0g; Protein: 0g; Calcium: 0%; Vitamin D: 0%; Vitamin B$_{12}$: 0%; Iron: 0%; Zinc: <1%

Storage Tip: Store in a reusable container in the refrigerator for up to 30 days.

Italian Hemp Dressing

Prep time: 5 minutes

MAKES 12 TABLESPOONS

Homemade dressings have an incredibly fresh taste that you just won't get from store-bought options. This dressing is easy to whip up, healthy, and versatile, making it a quick way to take the flavor of your salad to the next level.

- ½ cup white wine vinegar
- ¼ cup tahini
- ¼ cup water
- 1 tablespoon hemp seeds
- ½ tablespoon freshly squeezed lemon juice
- 1 teaspoon garlic powder
- 1 teaspoon dried oregano
- 1 teaspoon dried basil
- 1 teaspoon red pepper flakes
- ½ teaspoon onion powder
- ½ teaspoon pink Himalayan salt
- ½ teaspoon freshly ground black pepper

▶ In a bowl, combine all the ingredients and whisk until mixed well.

Per serving (1 tablespoon): Calories: 39; Total fat: 3g; Carbohydrates: 2g; Fiber: 1g; Protein: 1g; Calcium: 3%; Vitamin D: 0%; Vitamin B_{12}: 1%; Iron: 4%; Zinc: 2%

Storage Tip: Store in a reusable container in the refrigerator for up to 30 days.

Ranch Dressing

Prep time: 15 minutes, plus 1 hour to soak the cashews

SERVES 12

GLUTEN-FREE

This creamy vegan ranch dressing is oil-free and contains minimal ingredients but is packed with flavor. It's perfect for all kinds of salads or as a dip for veggie platters.

1 cup cashews, soaked in warm water for at least 1 hour

½ cup water

2 tablespoons freshly squeezed lemon juice

1 tablespoon vinegar

1 teaspoon garlic powder

1 teaspoon onion powder

2 teaspoons dried dill

▶ In a food processor, combine the cashews, water, lemon juice, vinegar, garlic powder, and onion powder. Blend until creamy and smooth. Add the dill and pulse a few times until combined.

Per serving (1 tablespoon): Calories: 68; Total fat: 5g; Carbohydrates: 4g; Fiber: <1g; Protein: 2g; Calcium: 1%; Vitamin D: 0%; Vitamin B$_{12}$: 0%; Iron: 4%; Zinc: 4%

Storage Tip: Store in a reusable container in the refrigerator for up to 30 days.

Lemon-Garlic Tahini

Prep time: 5 minutes

SERVES 4

My version of the classic tahini dressing goes well with so many meals—the options are endless. Try it with Baked Falafel (page 131).

¾ cup water

½ cup tahini

3 garlic cloves, minced

Juice of 3 lemons

½ teaspoon pink Himalayan salt

▶ In a bowl, whisk together all the ingredients until mixed well.

Per serving (¼ cup): Calories: 191; Total fat: 16g; Carbohydrates: 10g; Fiber: 3g; Protein: 5g; Calcium: 16%; Vitamin D: 0%; Vitamin B_{12}: 0%; Iron: 15%; Zinc: 9%

Storage Tip: Store in a reusable container in the refrigerator for up to 30 days.

Mighty Mayo

Prep time: 5 minutes, plus 1 hour to soak the cashews

MAKES 18 TABLESPOONS

Mayonnaise is a popular condiment, and this veganized recipe doesn't disappoint. Not only is Mighty Mayo creamy and delicious, it's also oil-free, making it a heart-healthy choice.

1 cup cashews, soaked in hot water for at least 1 hour

¼ cup plus 3 tablespoons unsweetened plant-based milk

1 tablespoon apple cider vinegar

1 tablespoon freshly squeezed lemon juice

1 tablespoon Dijon mustard

1 tablespoon aquafaba (the liquid from a can of chickpeas)

⅛ teaspoon pink Himalayan salt

▶ In a food processor, combine all the ingredients and blend until creamy and smooth.

Per serving (1 tablespoon): Calories: 46; Total fat: 4g; Carbohydrates: 3g; Fiber: <1g; Protein: 1g; Calcium: 1%; Vitamin D: 1%; Vitamin B_{12}: 0%; Iron: 3%; Zinc: 3%

Storage Tip: Store in the refrigerator in a sealed reusable container for up to 10 days.

Parmesan Cheese

Prep time: 5 minutes

MAKES 16 TABLESPOONS

GLUTEN-FREE **NUT-FREE OPTION**

This super simple vegan version of Parmesan cheese is a delicious alternative to store-bought products. Try it with Ricotta Red Sauce Pasta (page 156), Spaghetti and Meat-Free Meatballs (page 153), and Baked Spaghetti Squash (page 132).

1 cup cashews

2 tablespoons B$_{12}$-fortified nutritional yeast

½ teaspoon pink Himalayan salt

¼ teaspoon garlic powder

⅛ teaspoon onion powder

▶ Combine all the ingredients in a food processor and blend well until it's a rough powder.

Per serving (1 tablespoon): Calories: 53; Total fat: 4g; Carbohydrates: 4g; Fiber: 1g; Protein: 2g; Calcium: <1%; Vitamin D: 0%; Vitamin B$_{12}$: 6%; Iron: 3%; Zinc: 4%

Storage Tip: Store in a reusable container in the refrigerator for up to 30 days.

Substitution Tip: To make this nut-free, swap out the cashews for sunflower seeds or pumpkin seeds.

Turmeric Hummus

Prep time: 5 minutes

SERVES 2

RECOVERY   GLUTEN-FREE   NUT-FREE

Hummus is a vegan staple. It's delicious, easy to prepare, and makes a perfect dip for veggies or pita. It's also a great spread for sandwiches and wraps. As an athlete, I've always loved turmeric for its anti-inflammatory properties, so I brought the best of both worlds together in this recipe.

1 (19-ounce) can
   chickpeas, drained
   and rinsed
¼ cup tahini
3 tablespoons
   cold water

2 tablespoons freshly
   squeezed lemon juice
1 garlic clove
½ teaspoon
   turmeric powder

⅛ teaspoon
   black pepper
Pinch pink
   Himalayan salt

▶ Combine all the ingredients in a food processor and blend until completely smooth. Enjoy immediately or store in a reusable container in the refrigerator for up to 10 days.

Per serving: Calories: 472; Total fat: 19g; Carbohydrates: 63g; Fiber: 14g; Protein: 17g; Calcium: 21%; Vitamin D: 0%; Vitamin B$_{12}$: 0%; Iron: 34%; Zinc: 27%

Recipe Tip: If you want the hummus to be less thick, add up to 2 more tablespoons of cold water (1 tablespoon at a time) to the food processor and continue to blend.

Mushroom Gravy

Prep time: 5 minutes
Cook time: 10 minutes
SERVES 4

GLUTEN-FREE OPTION **NUT-FREE**

This recipe is great during the holidays or whenever your meal calls for a savory gravy. It pairs perfectly with Garlic Cauliflower Mashed Potatoes (page 118).

2 cups vegetable broth
½ cup finely chopped mushrooms
2 tablespoons whole wheat flour (or gluten-free flour)

1 tablespoon unsweetened applesauce
1 teaspoon onion powder
½ teaspoon dried thyme

¼ teaspoon dried rosemary
⅛ teaspoon pink Himalayan salt
Freshly ground black pepper

▶ In a nonstick saucepan over medium-high heat, combine all the ingredients and mix well. Bring to a boil, stirring frequently, reduce the heat to low, and simmer, stirring constantly, until it thickens.

Per serving: Calories: 26; Total fat: <1g; Carbohydrates: 6g; Fiber: 1g; Protein: 1g; Calcium: 2%; Vitamin D: 2%; Vitamin B$_{12}$: <1%; Iron: 4%; Zinc: 1%

Storage Tip: This stores well in a reusable container in the refrigerator for up to 7 days.

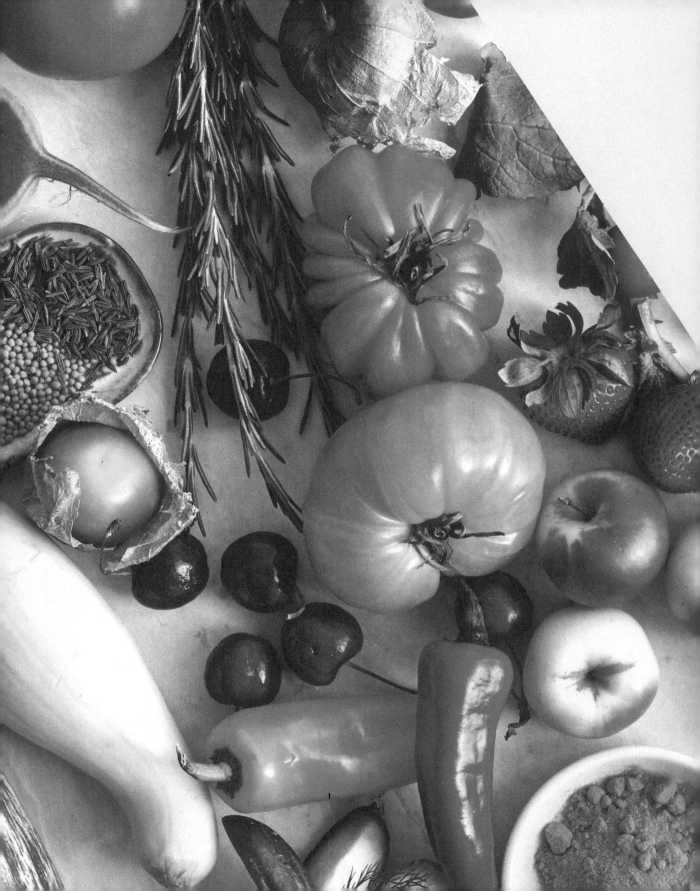

Essential Vegan Staples

Condiments

Apple cider vinegar

Balsamic vinegar

Hot sauce

Low-sodium soy sauce (or tamari, which is a gluten-free option)

Mustard

Salsa

Tahini

Flours

Almond

Chickpea

Vital wheat gluten

Whole wheat

Fruits (Fresh or Frozen)

Apples

Avocados

Bananas

Blueberries

Lemons

Oranges

Pineapples

Tomatoes

Grains, Pasta, Breads

Amaranth

Brown rice

Kamut

Oatmeal

Quinoa

Spelt

Whole-grain

Whole wheat

Herbs and Spices

B_{12}-fortified nutritional yeast

Basil

Black pepper

Cayenne pepper

Chili powder

Cinnamon

Curry powder

Garlic powder

Ground ginger

Ground turmeric

Onion powder

Oregano

Paprika

Pink Himalayan salt

Thyme

Legumes (Dried or Canned)

Black beans

Chickpeas

Kidney beans

Lentils

Nuts and Seeds

Almonds

Brazil nuts

Cashews

Chia seeds

Flaxseed

Hemp seeds

Pumpkin seeds

Sunflower seeds

Walnuts

Refrigerated Items

- Fortified unsweetened plant-based milk (almond, flax, oat, soy, etc.)
- Guacamole
- Hummus
- Nut butters
- Tempeh
- Tofu
- Vegan unsweetened plain yogurts

Sweeteners

- Applesauce
- Coconut sugar
- Maple syrup

Vegetables (Fresh or Frozen)

- Bell peppers
- Bok choy
- Broccoli
- Carrots
- Cauliflower
- Celery
- Cucumbers
- Garlic
- Green peas
- Kale
- Mushrooms
- Onions
- Potatoes, yellow and sweet
- Snap peas
- Snow peas
- Spinach

20 High-Protein Plant-Based Foods

Grams of protein per serving

1. Seitan – 63 g per 1 cup

2. Tofu – 20 g per 1 cup

3. Edamame – 18.5 g per 1 cup

4. Lentils – 18 g per 1 cup

5. Tempeh – 16 g per 3 ounces

6. Kidney beans – 15 g per 1 cup

7. Black beans – 15 g per 1 cup

8. Chickpeas – 14.5 g per 1 cup

9. Hemp seeds – 13 g per ¼ cup

10. Cashews – 12 g per ½ cup

11. TVP – 12 g per ¼ cup

12. B_{12}-fortified nutritional yeast – 11 g per 4 tablespoons

13. Peanut butter – 8 g per 2 tablespoons

14. Quinoa – 8 g per 1 cup

15. Almonds – 8 g per ¼ cup

16. Oats – 7 g per 1 cup

17. Sunflower seeds – 7 g per ¼ cup

18. Flaxseed – 6 g per 3 tablespoons

19. Pumpkin seeds – 6 g per ½ cup

20. Chia seeds – 6 g per 3 tablespoons

Easy Egg Replacements

(Substitutions per 1 egg)

Applesauce, unsweetened: ¼ cup

Aquafaba (the liquid in a can of chickpeas): ¼ cup

Avocado: ¼ cup

Banana, ripe: ¼ cup

Chia seeds: 1 tablespoon plus 3 tablespoons of water

Cornstarch: 2 tablespoons plus 3 tablespoons of water

Flaxseed, ground: 1 tablespoon plus 3 tablespoons of water

Tofu, silken: ¼ cup

Measurement Conversions

	US STANDARD	US STANDARD (OUNCES)	METRIC (APPROXIMATE)
VOLUME EQUIVALENTS (LIQUID)	2 tablespoons	1 fl. oz.	30 mL
	¼ cup	2 fl. oz.	60 mL
	½ cup	4 fl. oz.	120 mL
	1 cup	8 fl. oz.	240 mL
	1½ cups	12 fl. oz.	355 mL
	2 cups or 1 pint	16 fl. oz.	475 mL
	4 cups or 1 quart	32 fl. oz.	1 L
	1 gallon	128 fl. oz.	4 L
VOLUME EQUIVALENTS (DRY)	⅛ teaspoon	——	0.5 mL
	¼ teaspoon	——	1 mL
	½ teaspoon	——	2 mL
	¾ teaspoon	——	4 mL
	1 teaspoon	——	5 mL
	1 tablespoon	——	15 mL
	¼ cup	——	59 mL
	⅓ cup	——	79 mL
	½ cup	——	118 mL
	⅔ cup	——	156 mL
	¾ cup	——	177 mL
	1 cup	——	235 mL
	2 cups or 1 pint	——	475 mL
	3 cups	——	700 mL
	4 cups or 1 quart	——	1 L
	½ gallon	——	2 L
	1 gallon	——	4 L
WEIGHT EQUIVALENTS	½ ounce	——	15 g
	1 ounce	——	30 g
	2 ounces	——	60 g
	4 ounces	——	115 g
	8 ounces	——	225 g
	12 ounces	——	340 g
	16 ounces or 1 pound	——	455 g

	FAHRENHEIT (F)	CELSIUS (C) (APPROXIMATE)
OVEN TEMPERATURES	250°F	120°C
	300°F	150°C
	325°F	180°C
	375°F	190°C
	400°F	200°C
	425°F	220°C
	450°F	230°C

Resources

Animal Justice. Lawyers for animal protection. www.animaljustice.ca

Caldwell B. Esselstyn, Jr., MD. Prevent and reverse heart disease program. www.dresselstyn.com

Cowspiracy. Environmental documentary. www.cowspiracy.com

Forks Over Knives. Health documentary. www.forksoverknives.com

The Game Changers. Plant-based athlete documentary. www.gamechangers movie.com

Meat Free Athlete. Vegan athlete resource and community, including calculators for health and fitness. www.MeatFreeAthlete.com

Mercy for Animals. Animal rights organization. www.mercyforanimals.org

Nutrition Facts. www.nutritionfacts.org

Physicians Committee for Responsible Medicine. www.pcrm.org

Shirt Activism. Awareness apparel, with a portion of all sales donated to animal charities. www.shirtactivism.com

T. Colin Campbell Center for Nutrition Studies. www.nutritionstudies.org

We Animals Media. Animal photography, journalism, and filmmaking. www.weanimalsmedia.org

References

Alma, Lori. "Fat-Soluble vs. Water-Soluble Vitamins: How They Differ in Absorption and Storage in the Body." Verywell Health. Accessed January 18, 2020. verywellhealth.com/fat-vs-water-soluble-998218.

American Heart Association. "How Does Plant-Forward (Plant-Based) Eating Benefit Your Health?" Accessed January 16, 2020. heart.org /en/healthy-living/healthy-eating/eat-smart/nutrition-basics/how-does -plant-forward-eating-benefit-your-health.

Bagchi, Debasis, Sreejayan Nair, and Chandan Sen. *Nutrition and Enhanced Sports Performance: Muscle Building, Endurance, and Strength*. Waltham, MA: Academic Press, 2018.

Blomstrand E., J. Eliasson, H. K. Karlsson, R. Köhnke. "Branched-Chain Amino Acids Activate Key Enzymes in Protein Synthesis After Physical Exercise." *The Journal of Nutrition* 136 (January 2006): 269S–73S. ncbi.nlm.nih.gov/pubmed/16365096.

Campbell, T. Colin and Thomas M. Campbell II. *The China Study: The Most Comprehensive Study of Nutrition Ever Conducted and the Startling Implications for Diet, Weight Loss, and Long-Term Health*. Dallas, Texas: BenBella Books, 2016.

Carus, Felicity. "UN Urges Global Move to Meat and Dairy-Free Diet." *The Guardian*. June 2, 2010. theguardian.com/environment/2010/jun/02 /un-report-meat-free-diet.

Clifford, J., and J. Curely. "Water-Soluble Vitamins: B-Complex and Vitamin C–9.312." Colorado State University Extension. Accessed January 17, 2020. extension.colostate.edu/topic-areas/nutrition-food-safety-health /water-soluble-vitamins-b-complex-and-vitamin-c-9-312.

Cowspiracy. "The Facts." Accessed January 16, 2020. www.cowspiracy .com/facts.

Dombrow, Carol. "The Facts on Trans Fats: The Government Has Banned Them from Our Food. Here's What It Means for Your Health." Heart and Stroke Foundation of Canada. Accessed January 16, 2020. heartandstroke.ca /get-healthy/healthy-eating/the-facts-on-trans-fats.

EarthSave International. *Our Food Our Future: Making a Difference with Every Bite: The Power of the Fork!* Accessed February 12, 2020. earthsave .org/pdf/ofof2006.pdf.

Edwards, Terri. "Plant-Based Tips for Cooking Without Oil." T. Colin Campbell Center for Nutrition Studies. Accessed February 28, 2020. nutritionstudies.org/plant-based-tips-cooking-without-oil.

Esselstyn, Jr., Caldwell B. "Huffington Post Interview." Accessed February 28, 2020. dresselstyn.com/site/study10.

Esselstyn, Jr., Caldwell B. "Is Oil Healthy?" *International Journal of Disease Reversal and Prevention* 1, no. 1 (2019): 34–36.

Esselstyn, Jr., Caldwell B. *Prevent and Reverse Heart Disease: The Revolutionary, Scientifically Proven, Nutrition-Based Cure.* New York: Avery, 2008.

Fuhrman, Joel, and Deana M. Ferreri. "Fueling the Vegetarian (Vegan) Athlete." *Current Sports Medicine Reports* 9, no. 4 (July-August 2010): 233–41. pdfs.semanticscholar.org/9a77/5b05eda57eea8be2e037afe0 e9f984762476.pdf.

Greger, Michael. "Anti-Inflammatory Diet for Depression." NutritionFacts.org. Accessed January 16, 2020. nutritionfacts.org/video/anti-inflammatory-diet -for-depression.

Greger, Michael. "Optimum Nutrition Recommendations." NutritionFacts.org. Accessed January 17, 2020. nutritionfacts.org/2011/09/12/dr-gregers -2011-optimum-nutrition-recommendations.

Greger, Michael. "Plant-Based Diets for Improved Mood & Productivity." NutritionFacts.org. Accessed January 16, 2020. nutritionfacts.org/video /plant-based-diets-for-improved-mood-and-productivity.

Greger, Michael. "Skim Milk and Acne." NutritionFacts.org. Accessed January 16, 2020. nutritionfacts.org/2012/07/12/skim-milk-and-acne.

Harvard Medical School. "The Best Foods for Vitamins and Minerals: How to Ensure You Get the Right Vitamins and Minerals in the Right Amounts." Accessed January 18, 2020. health.harvard.edu/staying -healthy/the-best-foods-for-vitamins-and-minerals.

Harvard Medical School. "Know the Facts about Fats: You Need Adequate Amounts of Good Dietary Fat." Accessed January 17, 2020. health.harvard .edu/staying-healthy/know-the-facts-about-fats.

Harvard T. H. Chan School of Public Health. "Fats and Cholesterol." Accessed January 16, 2020. hsph.harvard.edu/nutritionsource/what -should-you-eat/fats-and-cholesterol.

Houghton, Theresa "Sam." "New to an Oil-Free Diet? Here's What You Need to Know." T. Colin Campbell Center for Nutrition Studies. Accessed February 28, 2020. nutritionstudies.org/new-to-an-oil-free-diet-heres -what-you-need-to-know.

Institute of Medicine of the National Academies. *Dietary Reference Intakes for Energy, Carbohydrate, Fiber, Fat, Fatty Acids, Cholesterol, Protein, and Amino Acids*. Washington, DC: The National Academies Press, 2005. nap.edu/read/10490/chapter/1.

Kanter, Mitch. "High-Quality Carbohydrates and Physical Performance: Expert Panel Report." *Nutrition Today* 53, no. 1 (January 2018): 35–39. ncbi.nlm.nih.gov/pmc/articles/PMC5794245.

Kim, Hyunju, Laura E. Caulfield, Vanessa Garcia-Larsen, Lyn M. Steffen, Josef Coresh, and Casey M. Rebholz. "Plant-Based Diets Are Associated with a Lower Risk of Incident Cardiovascular Disease, Cardiovascular Disease Mortality, and All-Cause Mortality in a General Population of Middle-Aged Adults." *Journal of the American Heart Association* 3, no. 16 (August 7, 2019): e012865. doi.org/10.1161/JAHA.119.012865.

McDougall, John A. "Plant Foods Have a Complete Amino Acid Composition." *Circulation* 105, no. 25 (June 2002): e197. doi.org/10.1161 /01.cir.0000018905.97677.1f.

McDougall, John A. "Plant Foods Provide the Nutritional Building Blocks for Optimum Health." Dr. McDougall's Health & Medical Center. Accessed January 18, 2020. drmcdougall.com/health/education/free-mcdougall -program/introduction/plant-foods-provide-nutritional-building -blocks-to-optimum-health.

Mero, Antti. "Leucine Supplementation and Intensive Training." *Sports Medicine* 27, no. 6 (June 1999): 347–58. ncbi.nlm.nih.gov/pubmed /10418071.

Moore, D. R. "Nutrition to Support Recovery from Endurance Exercise: Optimal Carbohydrate and Protein Replacement." *Current Sports Medicine Reports* 14, no. 4 (July-August 2015): 294–300. doi.org/10.1249 /JSR.0000000000000180.

Morton R. W., Kevin T. Murphy, Sean R. McKellar, Brad J. Schoenfeld, Menno Henselmans, Eric Helms, Alan A. Aragon, et al. "A Systematic Review, Meta-Analysis and Meta-Regression of the Effect of Protein Supplementation on Resistance Training-Induced Gains in Muscle Mass and Strength in Healthy Adults." *British Journal of Sports Medicine* 52, no. 6 (March 2018): 376–84. ncbi.nlm.nih.gov/pubmed/28698222.

myNutrition. "Nutrition Basics." Washington State University. Accessed January 17, 2020. mynutrition.wsu.edu/nutrition-basics.

Norris, Jack. "Omega-3s Part 1—Basics." Vegan Health. Accessed January 16, 2020. veganhealth.org/omega-3s-part-1/#background.

Norton, Layne E., and Donald K. Layman. "Leucine Regulates Translation Initiation of Protein Synthesis in Skeletal Muscle After Exercise." *The Journal of Nutrition* 136, no. 2 (February 2006): 533S–37S. ncbi.nlm.nih .gov/pubmed/16424142.

NutritionFacts.org. "Oils." Accessed February 28, 2020. nutritionfacts.org /topics/oils.

One Green Planet. "Facts on Animal Farming and the Environment." Accessed February 12, 2020. onegreenplanet.org/animalsandnature /facts-on-animal-farming-and-the-environment.

Oregon State University. "Essential Fatty Acids." Linus Pauling Institute Micronutrient Information Center. Accessed January 16, 2020. lpi.oregon state.edu/mic/other-nutrients/essential-fatty-acids.

Pearson, Keith. "What Are the Key Functions of Carbohydrates?" Healthline. Accessed January 17, 2020. healthline.com/nutrition/carbohydrate -functions.

Pereira, Marcelo G., Meiricris T. Silva, Eduardo O. C. Carlassara, Dawit A. Gonçalves, Paulo A. Abrahamsohn, Isis C. Kettelhut, Anselmo S. Moriscot, Marcelo S. Aoki, and Elen H. Miyabara. "Leucine Supplementation Accelerates Connective Tissue Repair of Injured Tibialis Anterior Muscle." *Nutrients* 6, no. 10 (September 29, 2014): 3981–4001. ncbi.nlm.nih.gov/pmc/articles/PMC4210903.

Pimentel, David, and Marcia Pimentel. "Sustainability of Meat-Based and Plant-Based Diets and the Environment." *The American Journal of Clinical Nutrition* 78, no. 3 (September 2003): 660S–63S. doi.org/10.1093 /ajcn/78.3.660S.

Ranganathan, Janet, and Richard Waite. "Sustainable Diets: What You Need to Know in 12 Charts." World Resources Institute. Accessed February 12, 2020. wri.org/blog/2016/04/sustainable-diets-what-you -need-know-12-charts.

Rogerson, David. "Vegan Diets: Practical Advice for Athletes and Exercisers." *Journal of the International Society of Sports Nutrition* 14 (September 13, 2007). doi.org/10.1186/s12970-017-0192-9.

Roza, A. M., and H. M. Shizgal. "The Harris Benedict Equation Reevaluated: Resting Energy Requirements and the Body Cell Mass." *The American Journal of Clinical Nutrition* 40, no. 1 (July 1984): 168–82. doi.org/10.1093 /ajcn/40.1.168.

Scarborough, Peter, Paul N. Appleby, Anja Mizdrak, Adam D. M. Briggs, Ruth C. Travis, Kathryn E. Bradbury, and Timothy J. Key. "Dietary Greenhouse Gas Emissions of Meat-Eaters, Fish-Eaters, Vegetarians and Vegans in the UK." *Climatic Change* 125, no. 2 (2014): 179–92. ncbi.nlm .nih.gov/pubmed/25834298.

Schüpbach, R., R. Wegmüller, C. Berguerand, M. Bui, and I. Herter-Aeberli. "Micronutrient Status and Intake in Omnivores, Vegetarians and Vegans in Switzerland." *European Journal of Nutrition* 56, no. 1 (February 2017: 283–293. doi.org/10.1007/s00394-015-1079-7.

Semeco, Arlene. "Post-Workout Nutrition: What to Eat After a Workout." Healthline. Accessed January 18, 2020. healthline.com/nutrition/eat -after-workout.

Shrink That Footprint. "The Carbon Foodprint of 5 Diets Compared." Accessed February 12, 2020. shrinkthatfootprint.com/food-carbon -footprint-diet.

Stokes, T., A. J. Hector, R. W. Morton, C. McGlory, and S. M. Phillips. "Recent Perspectives Regarding the Role of Dietary Protein for the Promotion of Muscle Hypertrophy with Resistance Exercise Training." *Nutrients* 10, no. 2 (February 2018): e180. doi.org/10.3390/nu10020180.

Thomas, D. T., K. A. Erdman, and L. M. Burke. "Position of the Academy of Nutrition and Dietetics, Dietitians of Canada, and the American College of Sports Medicine: Nutrition and Athletic Performance." *Journal of the Academy of Nutrition and Dietetics* 116, no. 3 (March 2016): 501–28. doi.org /10.1016/j.jand.2015.12.006.

Tufts University Health & Nutrition Letter. "The Pros and Cons of Frozen Foods." Accessed February 28, 2020. nutritionletter.tufts.edu/issues /10_14/current-articles/The-Pros-and-Cons-of-Frozen-Foods_1646-1.html.

U.S. Department of Agriculture. "Estimated Calorie Needs Per Day, by Age, Sex, and Physical Activity Level." Accessed January 16, 2020. health.gov /dietaryguidelines/2015/guidelines/appendix-2.

U.S. Department of Agriculture. FoodData Central. Accessed January 18, 2020. fdc.nal.usda.gov.

United States Anti-Doping Agency (USADA). "Carbohydrates: The Master Fuel." Accessed January 16, 2020. usada.org/athletes/substances /nutrition/carbohydrates-the-master-fuel.

United States Anti-Doping Agency (USADA). "Fat as Fuel—Fat Intake in Athletes." Accessed January 16, 2020. usada.org/athletes/substances /nutrition/fat.

Van De Walle, Gavin. "5 Proven Benefits of BCAAs (Branched-Chain Amino Acids)." Healthline. Accessed January 17, 2020. healthline.com/nutrition /benefits-of-bcaa.

Recipe Index

Subject Index

Acknowledgments

I am beyond thankful to my best friend and wife, Linda, for your incredible support and infinite love. Without you, this book wouldn't be possible. Thank you for always believing in everything I set out to accomplish. I am so grateful to spend my time on this planet with you by my side.

A huge thank you to my amazing mom, Elizabeth, for inspiring many of the recipes I've veganized over the years. Your unconditional love and support are things that I never take for granted.

Thank you so much to my sister, Eva, for always being supportive, trying all my recipes, and incorporating them into the healthy lifestyle changes you've made.

Thank you to my beautiful nephews, Joseph and Anthony, for always wanting to learn more about the vegan lifestyle with open minds and hearts. You both make me so proud.

About the Author

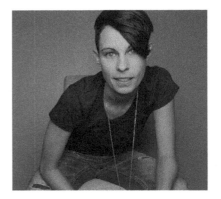

Anne-Marie Campbell is certified in plant-based nutrition and has been a competitive athlete for nearly three decades. She earned a black belt in Tae Kwon Do, and she's a hockey player and a former gymnast. Anne-Marie is a speaker and educator who is passionate about helping people successfully transition to the vegan lifestyle—for the animals, for their own health, and for the environment. In 2012, she founded MeatFreeAthlete.com, an online vegan resource and community. Thriving as a vegan athlete since 2011, she leverages evidence-based nutritional knowledge and personal experience to create delicious budget-friendly and low-fuss vegan recipes. Her approach encourages diversity and inclusivity in the vegan community, with a commitment to building a more compassionate and sustainable future.

9 781647 390181